WOMEN'S HAIR LOSS: THE HIDDEN EPIDEMIC

AN EXPERT PHYSICIAN'S STRATEGIC GUIDE FOR WOMEN WHO SUFFER FROM (OR LIVE IN FEAR OF) LOSING THEIR HAIR

SECOND EDITION: NEWEST METHODS FOR DIAGNOSIS AND TREATMENT

By Michael Lorin Reed, M.D.

LOCK & MANE
30 W. Bridge Street, Suite 2
New Hope, PA 18938
www.lockandmane.com

www.michaellorinreed.com

Library of Congress Control Number: 2012936345
ISBN 10: 0615622828
ISBN 13: 978-0-615-62282-8

Printed in the United States of America

Second Edition

Cover design by Mark Podwal, M.D.

ABOUT THE AUTHOR

Dr. Michael Lorin Reed is a renowned expert in the treatment of hair loss disorders in women. He is a board certified dermatologist and has served for 33 years on the faculty of New York University, where he has directed the NYU hair loss clinic and the NYU hair transplant clinic. He has been featured on *The View*, MSNBC, and ABC News Tonight, and has lectured and published extensively on the subject of skin and hais disorders. His most recent publication is the chapter "Hair Transplantation" in *Grabb and Smith's Plastic Surgery Textbook* (2007). His philosophy is that every patient is unique and thus deserves special attention .to their individual needs. In the end, it is about trating the patient, not just the problem.

Dr. Reed lives in Manhattan and New Hope, Pennsylvania. He has a wife, Margaret, and a one son and one daughter. He is an avid exerciser and advocate for the humane treatment of animals. He is also the proud owner of a red Doberman rescue named Marlowe Richard.

Question asked: *"WHAT DOES A WOMAN WANT?"*

- Sigmund Freud, M.D.

Question answered: *"GOOD HAIR!"*

- Michael Reed, M.D.

CONTENTS

DEDICATION

To my beautiful wife, **Margaret**, whose glorious and abundant red hair taught me the immense value of a woman's "crowning glory."

Her enduring love and sweet, but strong spirit have been my inspiration for this book.

PREFACE

I never planned to specialize in the treatment of hair loss. I went into dermatology because I liked to help improve the lives of people with life-ruining conditions like cystic acne or psoriasis. When I finished my dermatology residency training on June 30, 1978, I was not ready to go into full-time practice, so I joined the full-time faculty at New York University (NYU) as an assistant Professor of Dermatology. My main job was as a clinical investigator in the dermatopharmacology research section. We were involved in the early studies of new medications for many untreatable and debilitating skin diseases.

However, it just so happened that my predecessor, Dr. Fernando Stengel, had, for reasons never revealed to me, resurrected the defunct Hair Loss Clinic that some years previously had thrived under the direction of a professor I had had in the NYU Dermatology Department, Dr. Norman Orentreich. Orentreich is probably best remembered as the dermatologist who pioneered modern hair transplantation surgery in this country in the 1950s. Dr Stengel ran a rather busy clinic when his wife became ill and he had to return with her to his native country of Argentina.

I got Fernando's job in dermatopharmacology … and also his Hair Clinic.

So what did this mean? Well, despite the jokes people sometimes make about how it's great to be a dermatologist because "you can't cure ‘em and you can’t kill ‘em,” I was not of this ilk. I really like to cure patients. Or at least really help them with their affliction. I also like to get results rather quickly. For example, it’s very gratifying for me to find a potentially fatal skin cancer and surgically remove it. Patient CURED! Or to give a patient disabled by severe total body psoriasis a new medication and see him/her resume a normal, active life.

But in July 1978, there wasn’t much that we could do for all those women with Female-Pattern Hair Loss (FPHL) who made up the vast majority of clinic patients. Try to imagine being a psychiatrist with inadequate medications trying to treat patients with neurochemical imbalances. Not very pretty. I used to dread that Tuesday afternoon clinic.

So I guess that I can lay a claim that may be unique among hair loss specialists. I didn’t volunteer for this specialty. I got DRAFTED!

Fortunately, time has been kind to both me and, more important, to women suffering from FPHL. There are helpful treatments available, and women today can avoid much of the despair that dominated the clinic in 1978. However, despite all the progress we have made, large numbers of women are still frustrated in their attempts to find the help they need.

That is why I have written this book. It is my hope that women will read it and then help spread the information in both the general population and the medical community. When we presented this book to publishers, many expressed disbelief that there are really enough women with hair loss to justify such a book.

They don't realize that women's hair loss is the **hidden epidemic.** Unlike other health problems like breast cancer, you will not see women standing up in public to announce they suffer from female-pattern hair loss. They are too embarrassed. No woman wants to draw attention to her thinning hair. They fear that they would end up humiliated by ridicule and/or accusations of being shallow or vain. And that's probably true. It's okay to make fun of someone's hair since hair is public and private property at the same time. How many women would talk in public about their experience with breast cancer if they had to display their breasts? Don't expect to see a 5K celebrity run "to save women from baldness" anytime soon.

The purpose of this book is to make everyone aware of this epidemic, to give hope to those afflicted by it and to provide really helpful information on what can be done **now** about the problem.

INTRODUCTION

WHY IS WOMEN'S HAIR LOSS SIGNIFICANT?

The young woman was dying. Her emaciated frame looked almost skeletal after losing more than 40 pounds during her downhill struggle with anorexia. Finally she was hospitalized, but refused a feeding tube. Each day she was offered food and was told she must soon eat or would literally starve to death. And each day she would reply: she was fat ... she preferred death to her perceived obesity. When all hope was slipping away, she noticed that she was now shedding large amounts of hair. Someone who understood the significance of hair for women cleverly told her that if she did not eat, she would go bald.

Two weeks later – now 20 pounds heavier! – she was discharged from the hospital.

The above anecdote illustrates a real, core human truth: the importance of hair for females.

And so does contemporary history:

In the 2007-2008 Democratic presidential primaries, Hillary Clinton narrowly missed becoming the first woman in American history to run for the highest office in the land and most powerful job in our present world stage. Despite the momentous change in the role of the modern woman, the following statement was posted briefly by Mrs. Clinton in 2007 on her website HillaryHub.com: "*Pay attention to your hair, because everyone else will.*"

When a journalist wrote a piece describing Hillary in a blouse that revealed a minimal amount of cleavage, there was a great outcry and universal condemnation. Everyone seemed to agree that snide comments about female body parts should be off-limits in the context of a serious political candidate. But there were numerous unapologetic (and somewhat derisive) photo essays showing Hillary Clinton's changing hairstyles over time. No outcry. No condemnation.

WHY?

Maybe some clues can be found if we look into what is written in the holy writings of the three great monotheistic (and patriarchal) religions: Judaism, Christianity and Islam. Modern secularists often suggest that there are strong misogynistic currents in these mainstream religions. What role does religion play in promoting the significance of hair for women?

Seven hundred years before Christ, the great Jewish Prophet Isaiah wrote of God's judgment against Israel's Southern Kingdom (Judah) for sinful behavior, and women did not escape His wrath. Here is what their punishment would be:

The Lord says, "The women of Zion are haughty … Therefore the Lord will bring sores on the heads of the women of Zion; the Lord will make their scalps ***bald****.*

- Isaiah 3: 16-17 (emphasis added)

God knows what punishment really scores a bulls-eye!

The ancient Israelites (among other peoples of the Near East) deemed that the exposure of a women's hair to the gaze of strange men constituted a form of nudity and, therefore, was a temptation to sin. Long hair was also believed to possess magical powers among the Nazarites. Remember the superhuman strength imparted to Samson because of his long hair (Judges 16:25-30)? Covering the head of a married woman avoids tempting lustful advances from men other than her husband but has also been a sign of humility, respect and reverence for the deity (and maybe male authority?). It was, I believe, an act of creative ingenuity when the first Jewish woman convinced some old rabbi (probably her husband) that a beautiful hairpiece (*sheitel*) could be an acceptable substitute for the more traditional (i.e., less attractive and more humbling) cloth cover-up (*shmata*).

You go, girls!

But was the *sheitel* a Pyrrhic victory? Was it really still just a way to attract other men? And what if, ironically, the *sheitel* is more attractive than the woman's own hair? Pity the poor husband who tells his wife that she is more desirable in a hairpiece!

Christianity didn't result in any major changes in the significance of women's hair, although married women no longer were required to cover their heads when engaged in secular activities. Exceptions were those in full-time religious orders, such as female clergy (e.g., nuns). However, hair retained its special significance, at least metaphorically, as is revealed in the first question and answer of the Heidelberg Catechism written in the year 1559 (emphasis added):

> Q. What is your only comfort in **life** and in **death**?
>
> A. … He (Jesus Christ) also watches over me in such a way that not a **hair** can fall from my head without the will of my Father in heaven; in fact, all things must work together for my **salvation.**

Hair and salvation in the same sentence? That *is* significant!

Islam appeared on the world stage in the seventh century A.D. Hair retained its special significance as an adornment with the perceived magical power to cause men to lose their self-control. The traditional head covering worn in public was extended over the rest of the body, except for the face and hands. It should not surprise anyone that the subject is discussed under the title: **Preventative Measures** (Holy Qur'an, Chapter 24: Section 4).

Another way to establish just how important hair is to an individual is to look at the times and circumstances when people have been forced to shave their heads. In France after World War II, women who were known to have collaborated with the Nazis were rounded up –

and what was done to them? *They had their heads shaved!* This treatment served to both humiliate them as well as to identify them for further scornful treatment.

And what is one of the first things done to young military recruits in basic training? *They have their heads shaved!* This treatment takes away their individuality to enhance the process of indoctrination.

Why do Buddhist monks shave their heads? Because their religion teaches that it is undesirable for humans to pursue activities, including using physical adornments (i.e., hair), which emphasize individual uniqueness.

Another example of how significant hair is for women is what happened to radio personality Don Imus, who made his living by routinely insulting people with his sarcastic wit until he uttered his infamous last words by referring to a young women's basketball team as "nappy-headed ho's." He was accused of racism (the women were African-American) and subsequently fired. But the real *faux pas* was to ridicule the hairstyles of women with spiral hair texture that causes hair-control issues in a contemporary culture that regards long, straight hair on women to be very desirable. Retribution will always be swift and terrible for any man who makes fun of women's hair!

Finally, the value of hair has more recently been revealed by a short essay by William Safire in the *New York Times* on January 11, 2009, titled "HAIRCUT." The term is used metaphorically to mean "a sudden loss of equity or drop in income." Because of the recent economic catastrophes a lot of people and institutions have "taken a haircut." Hair is used here as a metaphor for wealth/money/income. Is there any doubt about the value of hair?

In conclusion, I believe there is something unique about hair that makes it different compared to all other physical adornments and attractants. Hair is the only physical attribute that is both *very personal* and *very public at the same time*. When a person (male or female) first sees a woman, there is initial gender identification along with some general physical observations (i.e., old/young, tall/short, fat/skinny, etc.). Of course, one notices how she is dressed, but clothes are not a body part. However, the first visible structure that establishes her as a unique individual is her hair. Other physical features such as the face are observed after noticing her hair. But HAIR ALWAYS COMES FIRST.

Finally, the significance of hair becomes painfully obvious to every woman who discovers that she is losing it. The blow to how she sees herself (self-image) and how she feels about herself (self-esteem) is devastating.

It is obvious that hair on the heads of women has never been there just to keep them warm in cold weather.

WOMEN'S HAIR LOSS: THE HIDDEN EPIDEMIC

1

WHAT DO WOMEN NEED TO KNOW ABOUT GETTING HELP?

This chapter is intended to provide the reader with the essential background knowledge needed in order to ensure the best chance of success in getting help for hair loss.

I shall use a Question/Answer format with YOU, the reader, as a healthy woman who has recently noticed more hair shedding than usual associated with some hair thinning. Your closest female friend doesn't notice a problem. Your stylist can't confirm it, either. So you see a local dermatologist, who tells you that she sees no scalp disease and no significant hair thinning, but she says casually that you could try the women's 2% minoxidil solution (over the counter). However, you've heard that when a person stops using this treatment, all their hair can fall out and that you have to use it for the rest of your life. No thanks!

The problem is gradually worsening and you are beginning to panic. The stylist finally admits that your hair is thinner. He says you should try taking vitamins. You think that stress is probably the cause, but your life is not going to get easier any time soon. You are now afraid that you are going to go bald. Should you start looking into hairpieces? You begin to wash your hair less often, but it seems to look even worse with less shampooing. You are having nightmares of people staring at your balding head. Anxiety attacks happen sometimes when you see other women with noticeable hair loss. Why are there suddenly **so many** of them?

The time has come to take serious action. You do an Internet search on hair loss in women. The search turns up a bewildering variety of products and services. How do you know what to believe and what works and what doesn't? Even interviews with medical experts give conflicting opinions about what is helpful and what is not. You don't want to waste your time on bogus nostrums, but you also don't want to endanger your health with powerful medications. And, you don't really want a hair transplant, right?

Okay, so let's work together and figure out how to move forward without making too many missteps. Your hair is depending on US!

There are five challenges, presented as "problems" that you must confront and overcome in order to accomplish your goals.

Problem #1 – How do you find an expert who can treat your hair loss?

This first problem is probably the most vexing one, because if you can't find someone who can both diagnose and treat your hair loss, you won't even be able to confront the next four problems. You are defeated *a priori* and might as well start looking into types of cosmetic camouflage.

You have already consulted with your stylist, your close girlfriend, likely your mother, and maybe even your husband or boyfriend. But, of course, you don't want awareness of your problem to spread beyond this inner circle.

Your visit to your local dermatologist was unhelpful. Did you get the feeling that she wasn't very enthusiastic about dealing with your hair loss? You're probably right. Dermatologists are trained to treat hair loss, but if you don't have an obvious *disease* affecting your scalp, they are likely to give you short attention.

Now you go to your medical doctor, or maybe your gynecologist, for a general evaluation. Your physical exam is normal and routine blood tests are okay. The doctor either didn't pay attention to your hair or said it didn't look so bad to them. You struck out again!

So who is out there who can do something helpful for your problem?

You could see a non-M.D. expert called a "trichologist." A What? Translation: Hair (tricho) expert. This "expert" is usually a transplant from the United Kingdom where there is some kind of specialized formal training (and credentialing) in hair and scalp care and nutrition. A good trichologist should be able to help you learn all you need to know about non-medical approaches to helping hair grow in an optimal way. They will discuss diet, nutritional supplements, scalp hygiene, etc. I believe that this information is valuable as long as it is not oversold as a substitute for the medical and surgical treatment that can be done only by an expert physician. I would be suspicious of any trichologist who has no working relationship with a doctor who can take over when non-medical treatment is inadequate, especially when the hair loss is associated with a disease. One good thing about seeing a trichologist is that at least you finally found someone who seems to have some knowledge of and interest in your hair loss. I expect that you might feel better than you did after your visit to your local dermatologist! But you have not accomplished your goal if you still have hair loss after pursuing optimal scalp hygiene and nutrition.

Maybe you haven't traveled this road yet. Unfortunately, it is a well-worn pathway leading to the final goal of consulting with a bona fide expert. There are a limited number of board-certified dermatologists who specialize in hair loss disorders. There is no hair loss specialty certification or official post-residency fellowship training. There are a number of medical societies that a dermatologist can join, mostly for the advancement of surgical hair replacement. Most dermatologists specializing in medical treatment of women's hair loss are associated with academic centers in large urban areas. You can contact the American Academy of Dermatology (www.aad.org) to find the name of a dermatologist who has been listed as a doctor who treats hair loss. The problem with this AAD list, however, is that any dermatologist can simply check a box on a questionnaire that says they treat hair loss and they get listed as a specialist. I examined the list and most of those listed in my area (NYC) are not hair specialists at all. And guess what? **I wasn't even on the list!** That's because I never bothered to fill out the AAD form.

(That has now been corrected, of course!) So if you call one of these dermatologists, don't make an appointment unless you verify with the doctor's staff that the doctor really does treat women for female-pattern hair loss, **including oral medication for female-pattern hair loss.**

You may also call the major medical center nearest to you and contact the dermatology department or division for a referral. However, I have seen patients who went to great lengths to see an academic expert, just to end up getting the "bum's rush" unless they presented some disorder of special interest to the professor. Unfortunately, seeing an expert does not guarantee kind and respectful treatment, or even helpful treatment. But it surely is preferable to no treatment or bogus treatment. At least you are likely to get an accurate diagnosis. But don't necessarily expect a warm, caring "hands-on" physician in this setting.

Another way to both get information and find an expert to see in consultation is to go online to medical education websites. At least half of my new women patients have learned about me from seeing me on educational webcasts discussing hair loss. Of course there are pitfalls here, just like when you go to see the professor at the medical center. Serious medical web sites carefully vet their experts, often finding them at, guess what? The local academic medical center! No surprise, really. But there are many imposters out there on the Internet, including quack physicians, who just are trying to sell you *something*. *ANYTHING!* Don't volunteer to be a victim. Sometimes hair loss makes an otherwise intelligent and discerning person very vulnerable. But that's what hair loss does to you.

False claims range from personal anecdotes ("I suffered from baldness and nothing helped until I invented product X. Now I have my hair back and you can, too…") to fake "research" claims that are unverifiable.

I am sorry, but you are most unlikely to solve your problem online. However, you can get helpful general information and perhaps identify an expert physician to consult with. I advise being cautious about buying products online that claim to **grow hair back** for women with hair loss. If they work at all, it is usually because they contain minoxidil, sometimes *al segreto*. And you can buy minoxidil (brand name Rogaine) without going to a "snake oil" salesman.

Finally, a simple first step might be to call your local dermatologist (or other trusted medical professional) and ask them to help you find a dermatologist who treats hair loss in women, including female-pattern hair loss. There are also endocrinologists (medical doctors who specialize in hormonal disorders) who might be able to treat women for hair loss and who may also know a dermatologist who treats this type of hair loss. Your medical doctor or gynecologist can probably refer you to an endocrinologist, even if they don't know a dermatologist.

There is obviously no simple or easy way to find the kind of expert you need to help you with hair loss. Patience, perseverance and tenacity are required to accomplish this goal.

But isn't your hair worth the effort?

Problem #2 – Why can't you get some useful medication?

Hooray! You followed my recommendations outlined in Problem #1 above and, after a few false starts, got an appointment at a major medical center to see a prominent academic physician with a reputation for expertise in the treatment of hair loss.

Filled with joyful expectations, you fill out a long questionnaire and are then seen by a dermatology resident-in-training who takes a brief history. Finally, the specialist comes into the exam room followed by an entourage of young doctors and a nurse. The expert looks quickly at the history, followed by a cursory glance at your hair and scalp. She exchanges a few comments with her fellows and tells you that the nurse will stay and explain your diagnosis and treatment plan. Then she departs with her minions, rather abruptly.

The nurse tells you that you have common hair loss and should try women's Rogaine. If that fails, you might consider a hair transplant in the future. Finally, she says that you can get a battery of blood tests, but not to expect any abnormal results. Lastly, she offers you the option for a scalp biopsy that can confirm the clinical diagnosis if you want it. You ask if there is any oral medication to take that might be helpful. The nurse acts somewhat annoyed and says that there is no "approved" systemic treatment for female hair loss.

You leave feeling worse than before you came since you don't want to use minoxidil the rest of your life. You also already had blood tests done by your regular doctor that were normal. You have no desire to get a hair transplant and are afraid that a scalp biopsy would be painful and leave a noticeable scar.

The whole experience leaves you with even less hope than before.

Let me explain what's going on here.

Welcome to the age of **legal medicine!**

Many physicians in practice today have been intimidated by the invasion of a predatory legal system, which doesn't distinguish between bad doctors who deserve punishment and good doctors trying to help their patients when something goes wrong.

This unfortunate situation has many ramifications, none of them really operating in the best interest of the patient. One result is that a diminishing number of physicians are willing to prescribe treatment "off-label," meaning using a medicine for a purpose other than its FDA-approved indication.

Off-label prescribing is legal, ethical and desirable for disorders that have either no approved treatment or inadequate treatment. The truth is that doctors know or learn about novel uses for medications years before FDA approval is obtained. For example, we were making special formulations containing minoxidil in the New York University Department of Dermatology to treat hair loss as far back as 1978, years before FDA approval. Our early endeavors were in fact the reason that Upjohn Pharmaceuticals decided to perform the studies that eventually put the medication on the market.

The bottom line here is that serious efforts to treat female-pattern hair loss (FPHL) require off-label prescribing practices. Only 2% minoxidil is FDA-approved for women and it is inadequate for a large number of these patients.

So if you are seeking help, you must not just find a doctor who has expertise in the treatment of FPHL, but must verify that the expert is willing to prescribe off-label medication, if it is necessary to help with your condition. The above anecdote about how frustrated you can feel even after seeing an expert is based on true stories I have heard over the years from numerous patients.

A deeper understanding of the advisability and necessity of off-label prescribing for FPHL is discussed in Chapter 4 (What is the medical treatment for female-pattern hair loss?).

Problem #3 – Why don't you just get a hair transplant?

There has been a widespread belief that women are not good candidates for surgical hair replacement because either their donor site is too sparse or the hair from the donor site will not survive long after being transplanted to the thinning area on the top of their head.

This belief is an example of how an idea can contain an element of truth without actually being true.

Yes, there are women who are poor candidates for this approach to treatment. Women with FPHL frequently have (or will get) thinning hair affecting their entire head (alopecia diffusa). However, this actual (or potential) situation does not necessarily disqualify you for surgery. First of all, the transplanted hair will survive the procedure and regrow for a long time, if not a lifetime. Also, if you are on medical treatment to prevent further loss, you may be able to keep the transplanted hair viable indefinitely. I have even had patients who had a poor donor site that improved enough with medical treatment to make a successful procedure possible.

I have not yet answered the question asked above: Why don't you just get a transplant? Now I will take it head on. First, you don't want any surgical procedure if you have a medical treatment alternative. It is the rarest of females who comes in wanting surgery as a starting point for hair restoration. This approach is antithetical to common sense. It's like saying you would rather have heart surgery than eat better, exercise more and take cholesterol-lowering medication. Right?

Another major consideration is that many women show up for treatment before other people can detect their problem. Of course, I can detect it and it is real (and distressing). However, these women desire to restore their original hair volume since they almost always have adequate coverage. Most of them are not ready for a hair transplant at this stage of hair loss.

The subject of when to transplant, what a transplant can achieve, who is a good candidate and the best techniques for women is discussed in Chapter 5 (What is the surgical treatment for FPHL?).

Problem #4 – How can a physician accurately assess your hair loss?

Let's say that you have been able to get past all the obstacles presented thus far and have had an adequate consultation. You now have a diagnosis and treatment plan and are hopeful that you might get some results.

You have taken the treatment for six months and return to your doctor for a follow-up visit.

The doctor looks at you, smiles and asks, "*How are you doing*?"

But you are not really sure how you are doing, except to say that there has been no major change.

So you say, "*I'm not sure, Doctor. What do you think?*"

She says, "*Well,* I *don't know. You have to tell me, right?"*

You say, *"Actually, I thought you would tell me. I mean:* ***you're the doctor****, right?"*

It's a Mexican standoff! Or maybe an exercise in agnosticism.

And what if you think you are worse? Can you really be the final authority on "quantifying" changes in your hair quality and quantity?

The answer unfortunately, but realistically, is **no**. Definitely **no**.

Why not? I mean it's **your** hair. Shouldn't you be able to tell? The answer is yes, no and maybe. Let me explain why your doctor has to have the final say on how your hair is changing with treatment over time with a true historical patient anecdote:

For more than ten years I have been treating a real patient who we will call "Sarah" for early-onset female-pattern hair loss

(FPHL). I have a standardized method of measuring both the pattern of hair loss and the degree of hair loss in the affected area on the scalp. Sarah had very thick and beautiful hair before it started to thin out in her early 30s.

Sarah was devastated.

Sarah started treatment and every six months returned for a follow-up visit. I would perform my exam and record my measurements before she was allowed to share her observations. I also never looked at my earlier assessments before the exam to avoid biasing my findings.

After one year of treatment, my exam showed slight improvement with a density score of 3.5 (explained below). But Sarah said she was definitely "worse."

After that visit, our encounters took on a repetitive quality. My exam showed that her hair loss, after that initial improvement, was stable. But at every visit, Sarah declared that she was unequivocally "worse." When asked if she wanted to stop treatment, she said that she preferred to continue in case the medication was at least slowing down her inevitable decline toward baldness.

Then, on our ten-year "anniversary" of her dissatisfaction with her results, a most unexpected thing happened. Here is the conversation that really occurred when I had completed my exam and asked her to share her observations:

Sarah: "Dr Reed, please tell me how long I have been getting treatment."

Dr Reed: "Ten years, Sarah. Why do you ask?"

Sarah: "Well, I have realized that my hair is the same as it was ten years ago so I think the treatment has been worthwhile."

Dr Reed (taken aback): "Wait a minute, Sarah. For ten years, you have been saying that your hair has been getting progressively worse. Please explain what you mean."

Sarah: "What I really meant was that I was unhappy because I wanted my original hair fully restored and it wasn't happening. But now I realize that my desire was not realistic. Actually, my hair looks pretty good. I get a lot of compliments."

Dr Reed: "Happy anniversary, Sarah."

I know that this anecdote may seem rather extreme, but it really happened and illustrates how subjective the patient's opinion can be. And that's perfectly understandable. Also, it doesn't mean that your observations don't matter. They matter a lot. But patient perception cannot be either the *only* or the *final* assessment of what effect treatment is having on hair growth.

I am now going to describe how I am able to monitor the response to treatment with reasonably reliable results. The technique has two components: *Pattern documentation and measurement* and *Volume assessment using a graded-rating scale*. In addition, these measurements are performed prior to hearing what the patient has to say and without looking at the results seen on any previous visits. This is called the "blinded investigator method" and helps minimize biasing observations.

The results are recorded on a diagram of the top on the head shown in the following illustration:

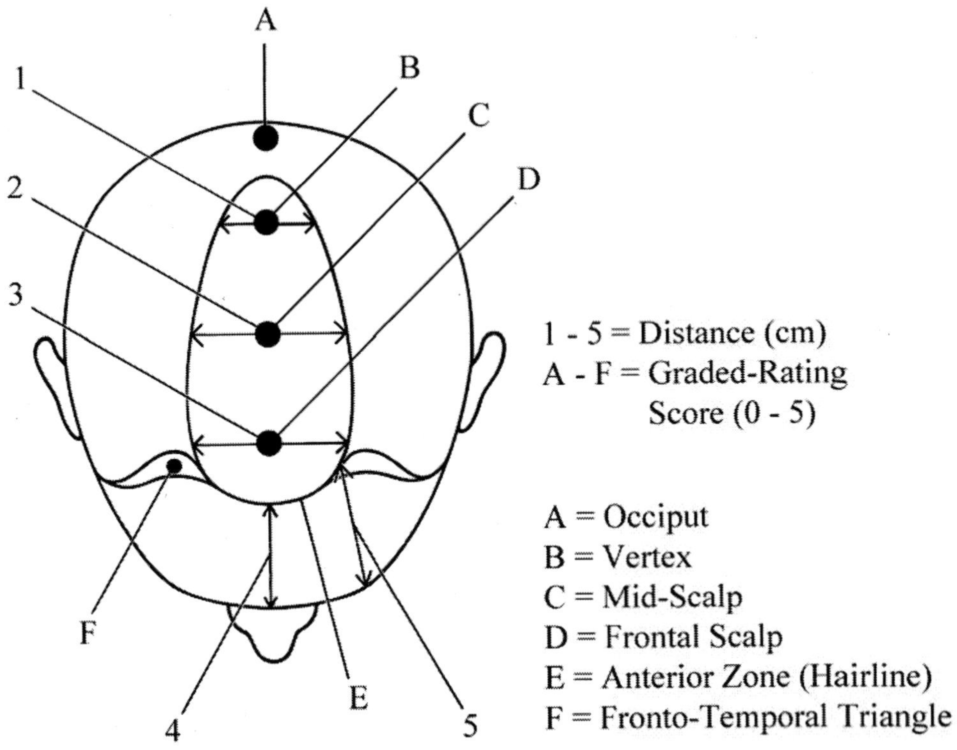

This illustration shows what needs to be measured in a typical patient with early female-pattern hair loss (FPHL). There is an area on the crown (top) where the hair thickness has diminished, resulting in the beginning of "see-through" hair. The side-to-side distance needs to be recorded for the three areas that comprise the "crown": the vertex (back), the mid-scalp and the frontal scalp. The location of the hairline at the midline of the forehead and from the lateral eyebrow(s) is documented. If there is thinning at the temples, it is given a graded-rating density score similar to the scores recorded from the three crown sites.

The graded-rating score is a five-point measurement interpreted as follows:

Score of 5 – Hair Abundant

Score of 4 – Hair Average

Score of 3 – Hair Adequate

Score of 2 – Hair Inadequate

Score of 1 – Hair Totally Inadequate

Score of 0 – Hair Absent

These scores are further divided to give three in between (sub) scores. For example, a score between 3 and 4 could be one of the following:

Score of 3<4 – Hair almost Average

Score of 3-4 – Hair between Adequate and Average

Score of 3>4 – Hair above Adequate

Most dermatologists are very capable of learning to use this graded rating scale if they are willing to make the effort and take the time needed. All they need is a diagram of the top of your head, a comb and a ruler. However, it takes experience over time to get good at making reliable and reproducible data. To put it another way, the technique is simple, but not necessarily easy. You are unlikely to be able to do this at home with the help of a friend or relative.

A discussion of what these quantitative measurements mean in terms of what treatment is desirable and what results can be achieved realistically is discussed in the chapters on medical and surgical options for female-pattern hair loss (FPHL).

Quantitative measurements can also be done using a more sophisticated device called the **dermoscope** or **folliscope**. This instrument provides an ultra-close up view of the hair shafts as they emerge from the scalp. The follicular openings (Ostia) can also be observed and may be helpful in distinguishing FPHL from other disorders. A digital imaging system can be attached to the scope and projected on a computer screen. A software program can measure various parameters related to hair volume. It is very impressive for a patient to see a close up view so she can better understand what is happening to her hair. However there are many technical difficulties when we try to use these high tech instruments to monitor treatment progress. Some devices (like the **Trichoscan**) require shaving and dying multiple areas. To find the same spot each time requires one or several tattoos in multiple areas. Patients don't like to have to do all these things and often refuse to allow it. And it's not right to bully them into doing it. In my opinion, such devices are best employed for clinical studies at the present time. A new device called the **Haircheck™** has recently become available that grasps a small clump of hairs and measures hair volume in a non-invasive manner. This device is potentially useful, especially with patients who believe they are getting worse when I can't verify it with my graded-rating scale. Although I have this device, I have not yet decided how to put it to its best use.

Problem #5 – How important and useful are objective tests in the evaluation and treatment of your hair loss?

Patients are very impressed with the idea of objective tests in every aspect of their health care and hair loss. It is a common scenario at the time of the visit for the patient to try to start with a discussion of the results of blood tests or a scalp biopsy performed elsewhere. Although this is understandable, it is actually an attempt to start the consult at the end and then have to go backwards to the necessary beginning.

Here is the main point I want to make: **The most important aspects of a consultation for hair loss are an accurate and detailed history and a careful, properly performed examination of the hair and scalp.**

I am not saying that objective tests are unnecessary, necessarily. But mostly they are either confirmatory or comforting by supporting the clinical diagnosis obtained from the history and physical exam.

Objective tests are also useful for the physician who isn't willing or able to spend the time and effort needed for a good history and proper exam, but who still has a desire to help (or impress) the patient.

Having said all the above, I still believe it's desirable for you, the patient, to know what tests are potentially helpful and when they should be performed. I am going to limit my discussion here to tests that are useful in the most common disorders. More esoteric tests may be discussed, when appropriate, in Chapter 7 (What about all the other kinds of hair loss disorders?).

The tests are discussed in the chronologic order where the opportunity to do them presents itself during a consultation:

(1) **The Hair Pull Test** – During the scalp exam, the doctor should grasp groups of approximately 50 hairs close to the scalp and gently, but firmly, "pull" through them as they are held between his/her thumb and forefinger. Hairs that are resting (telogen hairs) will come out "by the root." Up to 4 hairs per pull is considered normal. This test should be performed routinely to verify and quantify hair shedding.

(2) **The Hair Pluck Test** – This test is performed to determine the ratio of growing to resting hairs (anagen/telogen ratio). About 50 hairs are pulled out "by the root" using a plucking device such as a rubber-tipped hemostat. It is somewhat painful and leaves a small (and temporary) bald spot. Patients really don't like this procedure and will decline it when given a choice. It is used mainly in clinical studies to help determine if a medication is increasing the percentage of growing hair

follicles. It's not very helpful as an office procedure, in my opinion, and I rarely do it.

(3) **The Hair Shed/Pull Collection (Trichogram)** – Loose hairs obtained either during the performance of a hair pull test by the doctor or collected by the patient when combing/washing can be sent to a qualified dermatopathology laboratory for examination of both the hair shafts and roots for abnormalities or to confirm a diagnosis of Telogen Effluvium (Chapter 6). Microscopic examination of the hair roots can be very helpful in distinguishing between common conditions, less common disorders presented in an atypical manner and uncommon/rare forms of hair loss.

I find this test to be quite useful, but every pathology lab may not perform it. I suggest using the New York University dermatopathology laboratory if there is any doubt about another lab.

Another kind of useful information obtainable from a hair collection is to have the patient do a daily count of loose hairs found in the shower and in the comb/brush for ten consecutive days. These hairs are placed in an envelope with the date, number of hairs and wash/no wash written down. This can give the doctor a more quantitative picture of both the real severity of shedding and help to monitor treatment progress. However, it can sometimes backfire if the patient becomes overly focused on the daily shed. I have had several patients who, once they started doing these counts, became unable to stop. They probably suffer from an underlying obsessive-compulsive disorder (OCD) that finds some kind of relief with hair counting. This habit then takes on a life of its own and persists (sometimes for years) even if the hair loss has resolved.

(4) **The Scalp Biopsy** – This procedure involves excision of a small piece(s) of scalp from the affected area(s). The biopsy site is then stitched (sutured) to prevent bleeding and minimize scarring. The tissue is typically 4-5 mm (1/5 of an inch) in diameter.

A scalp biopsy should generally be done in three circumstances: (1) When the history and exam are inadequate to establish the diagnosis; (2) When it is desirable to confirm the diagnosis of an uncommon/rare disorder prior to prescribing potentially problematic medication; and (3) When the patient doesn't believe the clinical diagnosis and wants more objective data. The problem with scalp biopsies is that unless the specimen is taken from the right location at the right time, the pathologist is often unable to make a specific diagnosis. Instead, they give a list of possibilities that the findings are "suggestive of" or "consistent with." This kind of report is the best they can do. It's not their fault, but it's not that helpful or useful. In the final analysis, the clinician, not the pathologist, must put all the data in context to make the diagnosis.

I don't do a lot of scalp biopsies.

(5) **Blood Tests** – There is a battery of blood tests that I obtain from patients with common disorders to "rule out" potential underlying systemic conditions. If the patient has no other abnormal physical findings such as acne, facial hair, obesity, irregular menses, etc. (see Chapter 7), it is unlikely that we will find useful information from these blood tests.

Nevertheless, it is probably good to perform these tests at least once when you see a doctor the first time, especially if you are very young or have very severe hair loss. I also tell patients not to expect a "magic bullet" if they do have some systemic factor(s) contributing toward the loss. In fact, most patients are worse off, not better off, if there is an abnormal blood test, because it usually makes things more complicated and difficult, not simpler and easier. Sorry about that.

Following is a list of screening tests that can be done, although it is not always necessary to do all these tests for every patient:

(1) Thyroid Testing – Thyroid Stimulating Hormone (TSH), Free/Total T3/T4, Anti-thyroid Antibodies.

(2) Pituitary Testing – Prolactin, Luteinizing Hormone (LH), Follicular Stimulating Hormone (FSH).

(3) Adrenal Testing – Dehydroepiandrosterone Sulfate (DHEA-S), 17-Hydroxy-Progesterone.

(4) Ovarian Testing – Free/Total Testosterone, Sex Hormone Binding Globulin (SHBG), Estradiol/Estrone.

(5) Immune Testing – Anti-Nuclear Antibody Screen (ANA), Erythrocyte Sedimentation Rate (ESR).

(6) Metabolic Testing – Iron/Iron Binding Capacity, Ferritin, Complete Blood Count, Routine Chemistries.

(7) Syphilis Test (RPR) – Only if there is an appropriate context. What a relief to know your FPHL is not really syphilis!

If any of the tests #1-4 is abnormal, an endocrinology consult may be needed. If #5 is abnormal, a rheumatology consult may be desirable. If #6 is abnormal, a hematology consult may be helpful.

As a dermatologist, my job is to work on problems that exist on or inside the scalp/hair follicles. Since hair loss can be related to imbalances in other systems, I often need to coordinate treatment with other physicians, usually a gynecologist (for reproductive hormonal medications) or, less often, an endocrinologist (for metabolic hormonal medications).

Summary

This first chapter contains the basic information needed to get help for women with any kind of hair loss problem. I believe that if a woman could get her doctor to just read and implement the suggestions in this chapter, it would be possible to at least properly screen her to determine if she should see a specialist for further evaluation. As I have stated elsewhere, the only way we are going to make any major breakthroughs in helping you is if you can start a grassroots-type movement to initiate research in this area. Don't wait for the medical community to do it. It has to be from the bottom up, not the top down!

Now that you have hopefully gained some basic understanding on how to accomplish your goal of getting help and hope for hair preservation/restoration, we can move on to "Follicular Enemy #1": Female-Pattern Hair Loss (FPHL).

2

DO YOU HAVE FEMALE-PATTERN HAIR LOSS?

"My ponytail is half the size it used to be. This is not my hair anymore," says Melanie, age 35.

"I visited my dermatologist for a skin exam and she told me that I am losing my hair," says Patina, age 45. "It was a moment of utter despair."

"I always had a fabulous head of hair. Now I can see through it ... everyone says I'm crazy, but I know I'm not," says Christy, age 29.

Female-Pattern Hair Loss is the most common condition causing both thinning and shedding in the female population. A major review article in the prestigious *New England Journal of Medicine* on September 13, 1999 pointed out that the seriousness of hair loss in women has been grossly underestimated both in the mind of the general public as well as in medical publications. A mail survey done in 1999 using a 9-question postcard screener sent to 40,000 women aged 18 and older got a 48% return rate. This response was remarkable for an anonymous unsolicited query and revealed that contemporary research and development leading to helpful treatment is very underdeveloped considering the large segment of the population afflicted with this condition.

Despite the fact that this condition is very common, it is nevertheless quite complex and variable in its clinical presentation, differing patterns of hair loss, objective work-up and both its subtlety and outcome of treatment options.

How does FPHL initially manifest itself?

There is a moment in time and space when a woman experiences the terrible realization: "I'm losing my hair!" Usually, she makes the observation herself. Sometimes another person (mother, girlfriend, stylist, physician) is first to make the unpleasant discovery (at some potential peril for the relationship, of course).

So what is (are) the usual first finding(s)? Here they are, starting with what should be the most common presentation:

- Gradually thinning hair ("I can see my scalp.")
- Persistent hair shedding ("There is too much hair in my shower drain.")
- Change in hair texture ("It's not my hair.")
- Decreasing hair volume ("My ponytail is gone!")

- Decreasing hair length ("My hair doesn't grow!")

For many years I have asked patients to tell me if their hair loss *first* manifested itself as thinning or shedding - with very limited success. Most women say that they have experienced both symptoms at about the same time. They seem unable to pick one first. However, given the awful significance of realizing the onset of hair loss, it should not surprise anyone that multiple manifestations seem to occur more or less simultaneously. Indeed, many women notice some combination of several (or even all) of the above findings.

What exactly is FPHL?

The term Female-Pattern Hair Loss (FPHL) has historically been viewed as being synonymous with Androgenetic Alopecia. The latter diagnosis is defined as hair loss (alopecia) caused by a genetically programmed sensitivity to male hormones (androgens). Women make androgens in their adrenal cortex and the theca cells of their ovaries. Over time there is believed to be a gradual build-up of a potent local androgen called dihydrotestosterone (DHT) inside genetically-predisposed hair follicle cells, resulting in gradual hair miniaturization and a progressively shorter anagen (growth) phase. This process results in a gradual decrease in hair volume (see-through hair), and eventually many hairs stop growing and are no longer visible to the eye (vellus hairs).

This explanation for FPHL has been extrapolated directly from what is known about the development of Male-Pattern Hair Loss (MPHL).

But if this belief is really true, why don't men and women lose their hair at the same time and in the same pattern? Shouldn't there just be one disorder, perhaps called Human-Pattern Hair Loss (HPHL)? Men and women may at times appear to come from different planets, but their hair follicles are from planet Earth. The basic structure and function of hair follicles in men and women are identical. You cannot tell them apart under the high magnification of the light microscope or any other device.

Well, surprise, surprise! Hair loss in women is turning out to be more complicated than in men. Some authorities have gone so far as to say that FPHL and MPHL are entirely *different* conditions! However, I believe that most of us are convinced that androgens do play a significant role in both genders. However, in women the presence of high levels of female hormones (estrogen) in the circulation and the presence of an enzyme (aromatase) in the follicle that protects it by changing androgens into estrogen may help explain the usual (but not always) later onset of hair loss in women. Also, androgens must attach to a carrier protein called the *androgen receptor*, which transports them into the cell nucleus where they alter cell growth to effect hair loss. DHT is supposed to be the most potent androgen working at this level, but other androgens may play a role also and there may be differences in receptor-affinities in women versus men over time. Finally, the enzyme called type II 5-alpha-reductase, which converts circulating androgens to DHT in men may not play as great a role in women as men.

At present there is no adequate explanation for why women typically lose hair in a different pattern than men (see: How does FPHL differ from MPHL?, p. 37). Some investigators believe that FPHL is mainly due to a diminished effect of estrogens in the follicle and suggest we call this condition "low estrone alopecia". I think they have a point, but my present view is that there is an imbalance inside the follicle of estrogen/androgen that varies among women. Getting back the balance is discussed further in Chapter 4. Since androgenic (DHT) activity alone does not appear to be the only factor contributing to developing this condition, most experts at the present time prefer to use the diagnosis of Female-Pattern Hair Loss (FPHL).

Who gets FPHL?

According to surveys conducted by the American Academy of Dermatology, 50% of women will develop FPHL at some time during their lifetime, beginning any time after puberty. Twenty percent of women will suffer from noticeable loss. In the United States alone, this translates into about *30 million* women.

But who are the unlucky winners of the hair loss "lotto"?

We know that genetics plays a role here – like in most human afflictions. A common belief among lay people is a tendency for hair loss to come through the maternal grandfather, at least in men. I don't know of any epidemiologic data to either support or refute this idea. However, from 30 years of routinely asking if anyone in the family tree ever (tongue-in-cheek) "died from baldness," I can say that there is no predominant culprit(s). In my experience, somewhere around 15% of women with loss deny any family hair loss history in either men or women.

The simple truth is that we are just beginning to unravel the genetic code that predisposes men and women to hair loss. Some studies have found an association in men with androgenetic alopecia (AGA) and changes in the androgen receptor (AR) gene on the X chromosome. More recent work has shown an association between hair loss and defects called single nucleotide polymorphisms (SNPs) on chromosome 20p11. Further investigations will, no doubt, sooner or later unlock the genetic puzzle. But at present there is no way to predict who will suffer from hair loss and how severe it will become. Of course, if your family tree is riddled with balding men and thin-haired women … yes, you get it.

When doctors don't know what's going on, we like to say it using esoteric language. We may be ignorant, but we are not stupid! In this context, we say that FPHL is a *polygenic* (many genes) disorder.

When does FPHL start?

FPHL can start at any time after puberty. Over time, more and more women begin to notice thinning hair. There is no way (yet) for an individual to predict when it will happen. Many women appear to have some protection during their years of childbearing potential that is lost during the peri-menopausal (45-55 year-old) period. It is during this time that there has historically been a peak incidence of onset. However, that may be changing…

More and more women are showing up in my office with hair loss at an earlier age.

What's going on here? There are at least two explanations for this observation that are by no means mutually exclusive.

First, women in our western culture have over the past few generations expanded beyond their traditional domestic roles (which they still have) into what historically has been the male-provider function – i.e., working to pay the bills. Sometimes this increase in responsibility translates into a fulfilling career. But many women are forced to work to help the family survive economically. These women may simply end up with too many "hats to wear." There is evidence in animal studies that the stress associated with being forced to play a dominant role may increase body androgen (male-hormone) levels. Could these physiologic changes over time accelerate FPHL? There are no human studies yet to support or refute this hypothesis.

A more likely (and certainly less controversial) explanation is that women today are more highly educated than in the past and more visible in the workplace. Thus they are more likely to be knowledgeable about newer treatments available to them and more motivated to seek help since they are still judged by traditional standards of beauty, including having acceptable appearing hair.

Regardless of the reason(s), the trend for younger women seeking help leads us to the next important question that must be addressed.

Can FPHL be prevented?

At present there is no way to change a person's genetic program. However, it is possible to either accelerate or delay a genetically determined condition like FPHL. The following fictionalized, but very plausible anecdote illustrates this point:

Identical twins Jean and Jan were born 47 years ago. Their lives took divergent pathways beginning in the late teenage years.

Jean lived a very health conscious lifestyle. It was characterized by good nutrition, regular exercise, adequate sleep and moderate alcohol consumption. She stayed close to her family and had a successful marriage.

Jan was a wild one. Her lifestyle vacillated with unpredictable ups and downs. Her feckless behavior resulted in many physical problems and a number of surgical procedures. Her body weight often fluctuated up and down rapidly. Despite some close calls, she managed to survive and showed up at her 30th high school reunion along with her sister Jean.

One of the twin's female classmates named Sarah is a patient of mine who suffers from FPHL and thus is hyperaware of hair loss in other women. She reported to me that she was shocked to see a dramatic difference in hair between her two old school friends. Jean's hair was a little on the thin side, but probably only someone with a hair problem would notice it. Jan's hair was noticeable to everyone. Although her hairline was okay, she had "see-through" hair affecting her entire crown. Sarah was tempted to suggest that Jan see me in consultation, but was afraid to hurt her feelings.

The twins were identical no more!

This story illustrates a very important point about the development and progression of hair loss in women: ENVIRONMENTAL SENSITIVITY. *External factors* often affect the progression of FPHL and will be discussed below in the section on treatment options.

Finally, FPHL can be prematurely unmasked and accelerated by CONSTITUTIONAL SENSITIVITY. These are *internal factors* that include hormonal, metabolic, neurogenic, and immunologic influences. These factors are also discussed below under treatment options and further in Chapter 6 (telogen effluvium) and Chapter 7 (systemic disorders).

How is FPHL diagnosed?

The diagnosis of FPHL can be easy or difficult depending on the initial manifestation(s) and who is making the diagnosis. Generally, FPHL is either **self-diagnosed** or **physician-diagnosed**.

Self-diagnosis is usually made when the following combination of observations and circumstances prevail:

- Gradually thinning hair over the crown area beginning with a widening part.
- Only a mild to moderate amount of loss.
- No history of significant hair shedding.
- No history of scalp disorders.
- A strong family history of early or severe hair loss in women as well as men.
- Lack of any significant systemic illnesses.
- Lack of significant psychological problems.
- Lack of unusually stressful life experiences.
- Onset time in the peri/post-menopausal years.

Of course, there is a multitude of women who fall outside the above parameters. In addition, even women who accept the diagnosis want to know if it is the only diagnosis or if there is any systemic problem making it worse. And still others live in denial of the diagnosis because they think (incorrectly) that they have no hope because they "picked the wrong parents." These are all my patients.

Physician-diagnosis is usually made by taking a careful and detailed history and performing a proper scalp exam. If there is still some doubt that FPHL is the correct (or only) diagnosis, objective tests can occasionally be useful (see Chapter 1, Problem #5).

The patient must tell the physician when and how this problem began and then evolved over time. With some physician guidance, the patient should give all pertinent details of her experience from onset to time of consultation. This history may be rather long and even convoluted, but is necessary in order to not miss something important and because these patients really need to tell their story to a sympathetic listener who wants to help them. As the expert consultant, I must always be aware that FPHL is very common and may not be the only diagnosis (see Chapter 7).

The findings during the scalp exam will usually confirm the diagnosis and require documenting the following observations:

What is the pattern of the hair loss?

The earliest finding is usually a widening of the center part. Next, the area right behind the hairline begins to develop a "see-through" look. Gradually, the hair thins out across the crown (top) region. The part, which is supposed to be a narrow "footpath" becomes a "country road," then a "super highway," and finally, a "giant parking lot." In fact, the hair actually thins out over the entire scalp, but the loss is usually (but not always) most advanced on the crown.

Are the hair diameters uniform in the affected areas?

I use a specially made pair of lenses for ultra close-up observation of the hair diameters as they emerge from the scalp. I tell the patient that with these lenses I can "see things that no one else can see." This often gets a much-needed laugh out of the patient who asks me if that means that I can see her brain. Then I explain what I am looking at. I know that there are more high-tech devices for close-up examination on hair shafts such as the dermoscope that were discussed in Chapter 1, Problem #4.

On a non-balding scalp, all the hair shafts are close to the same width (diameter). In FPHL an increasing proportion of hair follicles begin to "shrink." This process causes a progressive decrease in the diameters of the affected hairs. The result is a decrease in hair volume/weight. This is the key finding, and is both necessary and sufficient to confirm the diagnosis of FPHL.

Is there a decrease in hair density?

A decrease in hair density (hair per square centimeter) is also present in FPHL. The thinning hair shafts described above are only part of the hair miniaturization process. There is also a progressive shortening of the growth (anagen) phase of the hair cycle. Eventually, many hairs no longer grow at all, but remain in a permanent resting phase (telogen). These are called vellus hairs and are only visible using the light microscope. On the scalp exam there are spaces between the remaining visible hairs that appear empty, although on very close inspection, they still have their tiny follicular openings (ostia). These are spots where visible hair growth has ceased permanently. I sometimes say that there are no totally bald persons, just people with invisible hair.

When are objective tests helpful with diagnosis?

In my experience, the most common reason for needing objective testing for FPHL is when the patient either refuses to believe the clinically derived (i.e., history/physical exam) diagnosis or needs further confirmatory data in order to feel totally secure about what's going on.

The following tests can be performed to further establish the clinical diagnosis:

Loose hair shaft/root examination – There should be no unusual hair shaft abnormalities and normal resting (telogen) roots (see Chapter 1, Problem #5).

Scalp Biopsy – Typical findings include: hair follicle miniaturization, decrease in anagen/telogen (growing to resting) hair ratio, and an increase in vellus hairs (see Chapter 1, Problem #5).

Blood Tests – All normal (see Chapter 1, Problem #5).

How does FPHL differ from MPHL?

A lot of women that I see in consultation state that they have been told they have male-pattern hair loss (MPHL). This is rarely the correct diagnosis.

It seems that a number of people (including even some dermatologists) like to simplify hereditary hair loss by calling all androgen-associated conditions in both men and women MPHL (or male-pattern alopecia).

This is more than oversimplification. It is also not true.

These two diagnoses (FPHL and MPHL) simply refer to the most common pattern of hair loss seen in each gender. The pattern seen in FPHL has been described above. And everyone has seen and knows the typical way men lose hair, beginning with a receding hairline, then an expanding bald spot and finally (in many men) the "cue ball" look with a fringe of residual hair on the lower peripheral parts of the scalp.

However, some women **do** have MPHL and some men **do** have FPHL. This finding has nothing at all to do with an individual's masculinity or femininity.

So how do we explain why these differences occur?

Well, I'm sorry to have to say that we don't really know why women mostly suffer from one typical pattern, whereas men are usually afflicted by another. And we don't know why sometimes the opposite occurs. Clearly, the inherent distribution of "doomed" hair follicles varies both between males and females and among members of the same sex.

One possible clue to help explain these different patterns comes from embryonic development. The hair follicles in the frontal scalp are derived from the same fetal tissues that become the facial skin. On the other hand the follicles of the top and sides of the head arise from the same primitive elements that give rise to the skin of the upper back. So different developmental genes may affect when and how hair loss occurs in these areas. For example, a woman may get the hair loss gene for the crown, but not for the hairline. So she gets typical FPHL. A guy might get the early-onset gene for a receding frontal hairline and a later-onset gene for loss on the top of his head. Further advances (through research) in understanding which genes cause hair loss and how these genes work to produce differing stem cell lines in different embryonic tissues will eventually solve this mystery.

Summary

Female pattern hair loss is the overwhelming cause of both gradual thinning and persistent increased shedding in the female population. In academic teaching centers, attempts are periodically made to open medical hair loss clinics in order to teach resident physicians how to diagnose and treat less common hair loss disorders. Invariably, the clinic is overwhelmed by women with FPHL desperately in need of treatment that is not usually available to them in the clinic setting.

Why can't these women get help in the clinic?

The answers to this and other important questions will be discussed in Chapters 3-5, which tackle the details of how to successfully treat the multitude of women afflicted by the "hidden epidemic" of female pattern hair loss.

3

WHAT IS THE NONMEDICAL (LIFESTYLE) TREATMENT FOR FEMALE-PATTERN HAIR LOSS?

1. What about delayed or non-treatment?

This treatment may be the most common choice (at least for older women) for a variety of reasons. Women don't go bald like men and when a woman's hair gets a little thinner after menopause, she usually attributes it to the aging process. In milder cases that progress very slowly, many women choose to do nothing beyond a change in hair styling. We all are accustomed to seeing older women with the prototypical "poodle hairdo" – short grayish (or bluish-tinted) hair with a tight perm. Have these women really "thrown in the towel" on hair as an adornment, opting instead for low maintenance looks? Not totally. I saw a patient recently who works in a facility for the aged who told me that when they have weekly salon day in the nursing home, the elderly women all line up for their hair maintenance treatment.

I don't expect many of these women to be reading this book, unless they are searching for help for one of their "other priorities" (i.e., a loved one) who suffers from hair loss.

2. What about diet?

It's always been a little scary to me that so many patients would believe me if I told them that their problem(s) could be solved by diet, vitamins and stress relief.

I wish it were really true. So what is true? And what is not true?

First, it is certainly true that optimal hair health, like all health, is best achieved by a lifestyle characterized by good nutrition, regular exercise and keeping a balance in activities and relationships.

Hair follicles manufacture hair shafts, which are made of protein (keratin). So it's necessary to eat a diet with adequate protein. I suggest high protein, reduced carbohydrate and low fat. Bad hair diets include those that are very strict vegan (vegetarian) or those that rely on excessive simple carbohydrates (sugar, bread, pasta, potatoes, etc.). Women must have some white carbs in their diet or they will go crazy. It is desirable to maintain a stable and optimal body mass without rapid weight fluctuations. Eating disorders characterized by starving, binging and purging are obviously very bad for hair growth.

3. What about vitamins/minerals?

B vitamins and minerals (zinc, iron, copper, manganese, etc.) are believed to play an important role in maintaining hair follicle activity that results in optimal hair shaft production. There are a number of vitamin/mineral/amino acid/herbal formulations available in health food stores and pharmacies to promote optimal hair growth.

My simplest recommendations for patients who want to take supplements are:

- Any multivitamin with zinc (15-20 mg)
- Extra B-Complex
- Biotin 5000 micrograms (5 mg)
- Iron as ferrous sulfate (65 mg twice a day) in patients with serum ferritin less than 70 ng/ml (ng = nanogram)

B vitamins and zinc are essential for hair growth and high doses of biotin have been shown to help reduce splitting of aging fingernails. Since the nail plate on the fingertip is analogous to the hair shaft on the scalp, it is believed that biotin may also reduce hair fragility in patients with thinning hair. There is also some evidence that patients who suffer from excessive shedding may improve if they can keep their body iron stores as reflected by the serum ferritin (the body iron storage protein) above 50 ng/ml.

4. What about botanicals?

I remain somewhat agnostic about the value of herbs such as saw palmetto, stinging nettles and African pygeum. These botanicals (plants), to the best of my knowledge, have not been shown to lower blood androgen levels in humans. There is one controlled study demonstrating that saw palmetto is helpful for patients with Male-Pattern Hair Loss

(MPHL). It is certainly possible that these plants could contain biochemicals that work inside the hair follicle to diminish the adverse effects of androgens (especially dihydrotesterone, aka DHT) on hair growth. I remain open-minded, but would like to see more extensive controlled scientific studies on botanical extracts (plant-derived biochemicals). For example, there is a parasitic plant found in India has been shown to have anti-androgen properties and may become a source for a future hair loss medication.

At the present time I tell patients that herbal supplements, to the best of my knowledge, are safe and may have some potential, albeit limited, value in slowing hair loss in some individuals. They certainly can't hurt.

5. What about stress?

Everybody believes that they have more stress than anyone else. Your stress is obviously worse than mine because it's *yours* and not *mine*. I tell my patients that they should avoid all stress. Then we have a good laugh. The mail survey mentioned in Chapter 2 found that among younger women stress was believed to be a major factor contributing to hair loss. I define stress as *CHANGE*: The more sudden, unexpected and distressing it is, the worse it is for the person subjected to it. Self-inflicted stress like the story of the twins in Chapter 2 (Can FPHL be prevented?) will undoubtedly make hair loss worse over a lifetime. Stress from uncontrollable events, like a severe and unexpected illness or a terrible accident, are unavoidable. There are many ways for us to deal with how we react to unfavorable circumstances. Each person has the choice to maintain a positive attitude ("with all this s--t there has to be a pony here somewhere") and to keep a sense of humor (if they have one, of course).

6. What about exercise?

I am convinced that exercise is the best single activity to ameliorate stress for a multiplicity of reasons. Let me explain.

There is a growing body of evidence that regular and frequent aerobic exercise may reduce morbidity and mortality from both degenerative disorders (heart attack, stroke, etc.) and many kinds of cancer. So how might exercise have a positive impact on hair growth?

First, there is the direct effect of sending oxygen and nutrients through increased blood flow to the scalp. The scalp has an amazing blood supply, which anyone who has ever had a scalp laceration will attest to. It has long been observed in situations where there is a persistent increase in blood flow, such as under a cast on a broken limb, that there is a noticeable increase in local hair density.

Secondly, I believe that exercise promotes a better balance between the metabolic system, the immune system and the nervous system. This is particularly important in females, who are more "finely tuned" than males due to their hormonal complexity. This is why women are so prone to episodic shedding (see Chapter 6). Men rarely shed. Hair growth is definitely influenced by hormonal fluctuations, metabolic activity and immunologic balance. It may even be affected by local nerve activity (neurogenic factors – see Chapter 6). Regular aerobic exercise has been shown to have an effect on the nervous system similar to anti-depressant medications. Individuals in great physical shape look and feel better, which can help them to deal with stress more effectively. I believe they may *suffer* less from hair loss. When a person is overweight and inactive, the thyroid gland slows down the metabolic rate of the entire body, possibly including the hair follicles. I think that it is possible to have normal thyroid blood tests and "hypothyroid" hair follicles. So I advise patients to engage in cardiovascular type workouts that last one hour, at least three (and ideally five) times weekly. I'm not talking about walking. Yes, studies have shown that walking is better than sitting. But I am talking about getting your pulse up and experiencing discomfort. Sorry.

For the record, my exercise advice is the least likely to be implemented, even by the most motivated patient. You, of course, know all the reasons (aka excuses).

7. What about hair care?

I am neither a stylist nor a hair chemist. So I have to be careful to avoid taking a dismissive attitude toward this part of my discussion. The truth is that optimal hair care is even more important in hair loss patients. We need all the help we can get to make our hair look as full and thick as possible. I have seen many a patient come in with sticky, unwashed and uncolored hair because she is afraid that washing, blow-drying and coloring her hair might worsen the problem. This is unfortunate and unnecessary.

(a) Washing: You should wash your hair as often as you need to in order for you to look your best. Thinning hair gets oily faster because the amount of sebum (a mixture of oil and dead skin) produced by the scalp is the same (or increased) so there is more oil per hair, resulting in a greasier/thinner look. In addition, the oil contains dihydrotestosterone (DHT) that might get reabsorbed into the hair follicles, possibly contributing to more loss. Historically, products sold to reduce hair loss have often contained scalp-degreasing (debridement) agents. Daily shampooing is fine, but labor intensive for some women. Every other day seems to suit many patients. I think that every third day is probably minimal. I don't recommend weekly washing for most people. For women who cannot wash their hair as frequently as I recommend, there are "hair powders" on the market that absorb oil on the scalp, which is desirable. Some of these leave-in products are colored to match your hair and have a camouflage effect that is also helpful.

There are a bewildering variety of "thickening/volumizing" shampoos, conditioners and leave-in products on the market. I am not going to promote one brand. Try different brands until you find one you like the best. These shampoos contain ingredients that temporarily coat the hair shafts and thus give the hair more volume/body. They are very useful.

Medicated shampoo is discussed in Chapter 4.

(b) Coloring: It's okay to color your hair as long as it is done properly. It's probably not good to frequently perform aggressive double-stripping procedures to make very dark hair into very light hair, which can result in hair shaft fragility and breakage.

(c) Mechanical Hair Styling: Mechanical texture manipulation (with and without heat) includes cutting, braiding, blow drying, Velcro rollers, hot combs/rollers, curling irons, crimping irons, flat irons, etc. The hot styling methods result in temporary changes in hair texture – i.e., frizzy to wavy, curly to straight, wavy to curly, etc. Blow-drying is okay as long as you don't pull hard on the roots. Overly aggressive mechanical manipulation can result in hair breakage in the short run (especially to fine or overly processed hair) and hair follicle damage in the long run (see Chapter 7). Braiding close to the scalp over time is particularly undesirable and can cause permanent hair loss (traction alopecia). I suggest avoiding excessive pulling on the hair shafts close to the scalp when using these devices. However, you can cut your hair any way that makes it look good. Longer hair doesn't result in any more hair loss than a buzz cut.

(d) Chemical Hair Styling: Chemical texture manipulation includes perming, straightening and relaxing. These procedures all involve the breakage and subsequent repair of the permanent (covalent) chemical bonds that connect the amino acids that form the keratin protein of the hair shaft. Disrupting these bonds makes the hair shaft soft (like putty) and allows it to be molded to a different texture before reforming the bonds.

Of course, if the chemicals are left on too long, the hair shafts may "dissolve," resulting in broken off hairs. One way to make straight, thinning hair appear fuller is to make it wavier or curlier. This suggestion, if made by the doctor, is usually poorly received by the female hair loss patient. She already knows this and, if she thought it was desirable, she would have already done it! Problems caused by overdoing these procedures are discussed in Chapter 7.

8. What about artificial or cosmetic hair enhancers?

Patients don't come to me for advice on cosmetic cover-ups except to get my opinion on whether or not these products will either worsen their loss or interfere with whatever treatment I recommend. I do not approve of devices that chronically pull on the hair close to the scalp, since they can definitely worsen every kind of hair loss. Also, it's probably not good to apply topical treatment to a scalp on top of a sprinkle-on or paint-on camouflage material as that may prevent the medication from penetrating into the scalp. I discourage patients from prematurely investing in hairpieces (wigs) since my goal is to make such items unnecessary. However, if they already have a piece that they wear on occasion, I tell them that it cannot "suffocate" their hair follicles because the follicle gets its oxygen and nutrients from its blood supply. I don't know of any product that is able to cut off the generous blood supply that feeds the follicles. If I mention a sprinkle-on product that is safe and useful, I find that patients seem to either really like it or really dislike the whole idea of it. Hair extensions are okay for increasing hair length and volume on the sides and back of the head, but not on top, please. They are expensive and high maintenance. They may pull on the native hair more than is acceptable and can cause breakage in patients with fine hair texture. Small clip-on type wefts may be okay on the top of the head for special occasions, but may pull on the weakened, thinning hair of the crown if improperly installed or overused.

Finally, there is tremendous variability in the quality and skills (as well as the ethics) of so-called professional people in the hair-enhancing field. Make sure to get a reliable recommendation before entering this arena.

Summary

I believe it is important to address the lifestyle issues that may relate to overall hair health for several reasons. First and foremost, healthy hair follicles are probably more likely to survive longer over time in patients with female pattern hair loss (and other kinds of hair also). Secondly, there is a wealth of misinformation out there and if I don't weigh in on this subject, I am leaving the hair loss patient at the mercy of every self-proclaimed "expert" out there.

In the absence of evidence-based medicine (see Chapter 4), I believe a common sense approach is the best way to go. And if you have common sense, you know it isn't that common!

4

WHAT IS THE MEDICAL TREATMENT FOR FEMALE PATTERN HAIR LOSS?

"I never used topical minoxidil because I read that it stops working if you don't keep using it ... and then you're worse off than before," says Karen, age 38.

"The pharmacist told me that finasteride is not for women. He said it has dangerous side effects and that I shouldn't even touch the tablets. Why did you prescribe it for me?" says Bernice, age 52

What are the treatment options for FPHL?

Chapter 1 outlined some of the reasons *why* women don't get help for hair loss. Now the time has come to discuss *what* treatment is available that may actually ameliorate FPHL.

First, I must inform the reader that this subject is controversial, to say the least. Women who research this subject will enter a minefield of conflicting points of view, even among expert physicians.

Why is this?

I believe the divergent opinions on treatment are best understood by explaining the concept of "evidence-based medicine." According to DL Sackett and colleagues in an article published in the *British Medical Journal* in 1996 (emphasis added):

> *Evidence-based medicine is the conscientious, explicit, and judicious use of current best evidence in making decisions about the care of individual patients. The practice of evidence-based medicine means integrating individual clinical experience with the best available external clinical evidence from systematic research...*
>
> *Good doctors use both individual clinical expertise and the best available external evidence, and* **neither alone is enough**.

So here is a dilemma. Anyone who tries to apply these idealized criteria before choosing any particular treatment for FPHL is likely (and justifiably) to conclude that there is no reliable therapy.

Why is there insufficient evidence-based medical treatment for FPHL?

There are several reasons for this, but the main insufficiency is a lack of available external evidence from systematic research. There are few large, controlled scientific studies (systematic research) for the treatment of FPHL.

FPHL is not a disease per se and thus is viewed as a mere cosmetic disorder by the FDA. Also, there is no systemic (oral) treatment at present that can be used in women of childbearing age who might become pregnant while taking it. The FDA operates on the perfectly reasonable presupposition that there are some women who will get pregnant while on treatment. There is no way they can be expected to approve medications for FPHL that could harm a fetus. I like to explain it this way to patients:

> *I'm going to tell you two things that the FDA and I agree on. The first will not surprise you; the second may shock you:*
>
> *First ... there are a lot of dopey people in this world ... okay, no surprise.*
>
> *Second ... THEY ARE NOT ALL MEN!*

The result of this unfortunate combination of circumstances is that no pharmaceutical firms will invest in systematic research since the FDA cannot be expected to approve the medicine, no matter how well it works.

So where do we go from here?

For physicians like me who must try to help women with FPHL, we have to move forward from the *ideal* to the *real*. The truth is that we can help women with FPHL, but we need to make some modifications to the treatment in order to proceed. There are several other ways to make treatment choices. They are as follows, in order of decreasing reliability:

- *Partial Evidence-based medicine*: Clinical experience and systematic research are available, but one or the other is inadequate.
- *Experience-based medicine*: Clinical experience is available, but systematic research is lacking. This experience may be either that of an individual practitioner or a consensus among multiple practitioners who treat hair loss.
- *Common sense-based medicine*: Treatment using sound medical judgment based upon general knowledge of human hair biology.
- *Anecdote-based medicine*: Treatment based upon credible individual testimonials. An intelligent and reliable patient who took a medication for some condition that unexpectedly appeared to help hair grow would be an example. Stories from Internet chat rooms or from people peddling hair products are usually unreliable.

Following is an outline of treatment options for FPHL:

1. Topical/Local treatment.
2. Systemic (oral) treatment.
3. Combination (topical/systemic) treatment.

1. Topical/Local Treatment (evidence, partial evidence and experience-based advice)

"I tried minoxidil and it didn't work. I didn't see any new hair growth after three whole months! It was too messy to use in

the morning, but I put it on at bedtime at least every other night. I think it was a waste of time," says Jillian, age 33.

Topical minoxidil (evidence-based and experience-based)

We have been using minoxidil since at least 1978 to enhance hair growth after the drug was found to cause widespread increased body hair (hypertrichosis) when given orally as a high blood pressure medication. Locally applied minoxidil solution is FDA-approved and readily available over the counter (OTC) in both 2% and 5% concentrations. The 2% product is approved for both men and women and the 5% is approved for men, although women can legally buy it and use it. It is available as either generic (minoxidil) or brand (Rogaine). There is also a newer foam-base Rogaine brand. It is less irritating than the solution, but more difficult to get into the scalp for patients with early thinning.

I have always believed that Rogaine (minoxidil) should have been called "Retaine" since significant hair regrowth is achieved mostly in the vertex area, which doesn't thrill patients who are usually looking for more hair on their frontal scalp. However, it definitely does slow down and, in some cases, arrest further loss if used properly. The best results in women are usually achieved by "thickening" the hair shafts on their crown which causes a narrowing of the "widened" part in both the mid and posterior scalp areas. These are happy patients. However, any treatment for hair loss, including minoxidil, must be used for at least six months (and ideally a full year) before concluding that it is not helpful. Putting a solution on the scalp twice daily for a year without seeing rapid and significant hair regrowth is beyond the capacity of many individuals. But negative testimonies like Jillian's (above) usually result from improper expectations or inadequate use of this very helpful medication.

Low-Level Laser Therapy (LLLT) (partial evidence-based)

Low-level laser therapy (LLLT) has been used for many years to enhance wound healing. These devices are also called cold lasers since they do not burn or otherwise damage the skin. For the past 10 years they have been studied and marketed to treat hair loss.

The devices come in three general types: (1) A dome-shaped apparatus (LDS 100) placed over the scalp of the patient in a hair salon-type setting; (2) Several variations of hand-held devices for home use. Treatment is recommended for 15-30 minutes, 2 or 3 times a week for a period of 6-12 months to determine efficacy; (3) A newer LASERCAP™ that is worn inside a hat, such as a baseball cap with a portable and rechargeable battery pack that allows the user to move about with hands free. This "cap" covers the entire crown and is considerably more powerful than the other devices. I purchased one a year ago to try out and have seen a definite improvement in my overall hair volume. I am cautiously optimistic that, if LLLT is helpful for hair loss, this might be the best one so far, but the jury is still out. Patients can only purchase the cap through a physician's office at the present time.

The exact mechanism of action of LLLT is not known. It is believed that the laser energy may work by increasing the local microcirculation (i.e., oxygen and nutrients) or might stimulate intracellular mitochondria (the energy producers) to increase the size of the hair follicle cells and, by extension, the resulting hair shaft diameters.

At present, I tell my patients that I think LLLT has a place in our therapeutic armamentarium as an *adjunctive* (i.e., accessory) therapy along with proven medical/surgical treatments. However, I would be happy to have patients try the laser alone for 6-12 months if they volunteer (and don't mind buying one). Unfortunately, patients seen in consultation don't want to do this and rightfully expect to be given the treatment that has proven to be worthwhile in my experience. I would like to see a large-scale independent controlled study to find out exactly how efficacious LLLT is really.

Special Formulations (experience-based and anecdotal-based)

Since the FDA does not regulate the doctor's office, there is a long tradition of providing special treatment formulations. These are preparations that your physician believes are helpful, but have not yet gone through the laborious (and expensive) process of FDA approval in order for them to be available in pharmacies. For hair loss patients these formulations are usually topical lotions containing some combination of three elements: (1) A special *vehicle*; (2) a higher *concentration* of minoxidil than what is in OTC products; and (3) additional *active ingredients* that may enhance hair growth.

The vehicle is the solution that the active ingredient is dissolved in so that it can penetrate the scalp and reach the growing part of the hair follicle. If the active component is either not in solution or doesn't get to the hair follicle, it will not work. Unfortunately, minoxidil is not soluble in water alone. Propylene glycol is the solvent that is used in all the OTC minoxidil solutions. It has a somewhat oily consistency and is irritating in higher concentrations. The 2% solution has 20% propylene glycol and the 5% solution contains 50%. The 2% formulation is usually tolerated, but the 5% is often too irritating to the scalp. Also, some patients are actually allergic to propylene glycol. For these reasons I have several propylene glycol-free vehicles available that are usually well tolerated.

Concentrations higher than 5% can be achieved using these special vehicles. However, it is difficult to get concentrations above 6-7% in a vehicle that will not be too irritating when applied to the scalp. Some doctors claim to have up to 15% in solution, but I doubt whether this is possible, and I do not believe concentrations at this level do any better than 6-7%. Experience has demonstrated that the higher strength formulations can be used once daily, which is much easier than the twice a day recommendations for OTC minoxidil.

A somewhat bewildering variety of extra ingredients have been added to minoxidil preparations. The non-medical list includes vitamins, amino acids, minerals and herbs. I don't know if such ingredients are really helpful or not. However, I do believe that there are some medications that are potentially beneficial for selected patients. I generally prefer to use straight minoxidil with or without systemic treatment (see below) most of the time since the results are more predicable based upon use experience. However, if a patient fails to respond to (or tolerate) more conventional treatment, we can "add" active medications such as **ketoconazole** (see below) or **dutasteride** (a reductase enzyme inhibitor). Also, I can add retinoic acid to enhance minoxidil penetration or **triamcinolone acetonide** (a type of cortisone) to reduce scalp irritation, if needed.

The most recent extra ingredient that I am adding to the special minoxidil formulation is estrone in a low concentration (0.05%). This is based on the evolving concept that FPHL is often, if not always, caused by a hormonal imbalance inside hair follicles. There is too much androgen (male hormone) influence and too little estrogen (female hormone). We know that during pregnancy hair grows well due to high body estrogen levels. Adding estrogen to a locally applied formulation is an attempt to "fool" the hair follicles into thinking they are "pregnant" without fooling the rest of the body, thus avoiding risks of systemic exposure. At the 2010 meeting of the International Hair Restoration Society, the concept of "low estrone alopecia" was presented and it was reported that estrone has been used safely and with success in FPHL patients. However, to be on safe ground here, I do obtain baseline estrone levels in patients who may wish to use this treatment. How well it works remains to be seen, but I am optimistic about it.

Ketoconazole (partial-evidence based)

Ketoconazole is an antifungal medication that is available in the form of pills, topical cream/gel, and shampoos (1% OTC and 2% prescription-strength). The main use in the dermatology population is to treat seborrheic dermatitis and various fungus/yeast infections. However, there is some limited study data suggesting it may be as effective as 2% minoxidil. Some researchers believe it may help reduce DHT scalp levels when used with oral finasteride (see below). It has an anti-inflammatory effect that might also make it useful in patients with hair loss disorders discussed in Chapter 7. I don't know of any studies demonstrating its use as a topical cream/gel to treat hair loss. However, if a shampoo is useful, a leave-in preparation should be even better. That is the rationale for adding it to our special minoxidil formulation. It has not, to my knowledge, been used orally to treat hair loss because of potential adverse effects on the liver and adrenal gland.

2. Systemic treatment (partial-evidence and experience-based advice)

Oral medication is limited and controversial as discussed earlier in this chapter. However, it is desirable and very useful for a large percentage of patients seen in consultation by dermatologists who treat female-pattern hair loss. I am going to confine my discussion here to medications that are available in the USA and which have been shown to be helpful based upon clinical experience with or without support by published scientific studies. There are three types of oral medication that are recognized to be potentially useful to treat FPHL. They are: (1) some **oral contraceptives/ hormone replacement therapies**; (2) **5-alpha-reductase enzyme blockers**; and (3) **androgen receptor blockers**.

Women have great hair during pregnancy. Oral contraceptives "fool" the body into thinking it is pregnant. So we might expect hair to grow better if the patient is on some type of oral contraceptive. Higher estrogen pills are best if they are tolerated and safe for the patient. Also, the progestin component can assist if it has androgen-blocking potential. An example of a pill of this type is Yasmin, which contains 30 micrograms of estrogen and a progestin called drospirenone, which has anti-androgen properties similar to spironolactone (see below). I generally prefer to involve the patient's gynecologist since she must monitor a patient on oral contraceptives. The same applies to hormone replacement therapy (HRT) for post-menopausal women. I generally tell patients that if it is desirable and safe to be on HRT for unpleasant symptoms related to menopause, their hair may also benefit. However, as a dermatologist, I allow the gynecologist to have the final say on this type of treatment.

The only medication in common use in the USA that is used as an androgen receptor blocker is spironolactone (brand name Aldactone). This drug is classified as a weak potassium-sparing diuretic used with medications for high blood pressure. It is also used off-label for adult female acne and hirsutism (excess facial hair). This drug reduces androgen production in the adrenal glands and blocks the ability of male hormones to get into the nucleus of hair follicle cells. I do not use it in very elderly women or anyone with serious chronic diseases like diabetes mellitus, chronic kidney/cardiac disease and hypertension without careful monitoring of blood potassium levels. Healthy patients are told to avoid dietary supplements including potassium-containing salt substitutes and certain potassium-rich herbs, including stinging nettles (urtica dioica) sometimes used as a botanical hair supplement. Finally, non-steroidal anti-inflammatory drugs like ibuprofen can potentially increase potassium levels if taken in large doses with spironolactone. Lastly, oral ketoconazole can do the same thing, but we haven't thus far used it for hair loss. Topical ketoconazole should not be a problem. Spironolactone probably works best in women with systemic hyperandrogen disorders such as polycystic ovarian syndrome discussed in Chapter 7. It is the first choice of many hair loss specialists for a systemic medication, probably because it has been around a long time as a diuretic that pharmacists are accustomed to dispensing. So they don't tell the patient it is only for men as they often do with the enzyme blockers discussed next. However, like the enzyme blockers, it must not be given to women of childbearing age who might become pregnant while taking it due to the risk of feminizing a male fetus.

In my experience, spironolactone, given in doses adequate for hair loss (100-200 mg daily), is less well tolerated than the enzyme blockers. It is similar to oral contraception in its tolerability.

The final type of medications are the 5 alpha-reductase enzyme blockers, which include finasteride 1 mg (brand name Propecia), finasteride 5mg (brand name Proscar) and dutasteride 0.5 mg (brand name Avodart). These drugs are used to treat male-pattern hair loss (MPHL) and benign prostatic hypertrophy (BPH). They block the production of dihydrotestosterone (DHT) in both the scalp and the liver. DHT plays a major role in MPHL and is believed to also contribute to the development of FPHL, albeit to a lesser extent. Proscar has been shown in published studies of women to be useful in the treatment of hirsutism and is also safe because it doesn't change the ratio of estrogen to androgen. There may be a slight increase in both estradiol and testosterone in the body, but values remain well within the normal range. Of course, as with every systemic medication, a woman of childbearing potential should not take these medications if she may become pregnant while on treatment.

In my experience, the enzyme blockers are the most well tolerated systemic treatments. The main problem, however, is that they are only approved for men with hair loss (Propecia) and BPH (Proscar and Avodart). So when a woman presents a prescription to some pharmacists, they are told that it is only for men and that women "don't use it," "can't use it," "shouldn't use it," etc. Some pharmacists may even refuse to fill the prescription for fear of being sued by the patient if she gets pregnant.

For the record, it is customary for a pharmacist to fill prescriptions for off-label uses, if they are written by a knowledgeable physician with special expertise.

Finally, there was a small study performed on 137 post-menopausal females for one year comparing Propecia (1 mg finasteride) to a placebo that showed no statistical difference on hair regrowth. This is because this dose is too low for this age group and was probably given for too short a time. Women in this age group need the 5 mg dose of finasteride. Younger women may do alright with a lower dose, depending on how severe their condition is when starting treatment. A more recent study from Italy supports the safety and efficacy of finasteride for FPHL. 36 of 37 women of childbearing potential experienced no further hair loss and 60% had more hair after one year on 2 ½ mg of finasteride daily while also on Yasmin for contraception. Unfortunately, there was no Yasmin control group. However, these statistics are very similar to my clinical experience over many years with this patient population.

There may be a new breakthrough in predicting which women have FPHL that is androgenic and responsive to systemic anti-androgens such as finasteride or spironolactone. A biotech lab can now perform a DNA test that measures the length of the androgen-receptor gene, which is located on the X-chromosome. Women with a shorter gene are much more likely to obtain noticeable hair regrowth than those with a longer gene. We are now doing this test on new patients who want to know how likely they are to get desirable results.

The test is done on tissue obtained by a simple swabbing of the buccal mucosa inside the mouth.

3. Combination (topical/systemic) treatment (partial evidence and experience-based advice)

It is a common practice among hair loss physicians to employ multiple treatment modalities for the FPHL patient from the get go. Usually, I combine some form of topical minoxidil with one or more of the oral medications depending upon the age of the patient and the degree of hair loss at the initial visit. It is also customary to have the patient on some type of oral contraceptive, ideally an estrogen-dominant one, if I prescribe either an enzyme or receptor blocker. If the patient is unable to take Yasmin (or equivalent), I suggest she consult with her gynecologist to get one with low androgen activity.

I rarely start a patient on both finasteride and spironolactone at the same time. It is not usually necessary, but I will do it if there is an inadequate response to monotherapy (one medication). It is easier and less potentially problematic to use sequential treatment. As in doing math, it's easier to add than to subtract. The minimal treatment that will obtain an optimal effect is the wisest choice.

Patients also sometimes express a strong preference for one form of treatment over another. Some individuals just cannot or will not use topical treatment due to either the inconvenience or how it makes their hair look. Another group has an aversion to oral medication that is usually based upon a lack of understanding of pharmacology (how drugs work in the body). Of course, there are some patients, usually in poor health on multiple medications, in which systemic treatment is not advisable. Ironically, the vast numbers of calls about treatment side effects are related to topical, rather than systemic medication (see below).

I would ideally prefer to employ monotherapy, either topical or oral, for every patient. However, many of the women I see have lost so much hair or are so distraught about it that a combination of topical and oral treatment is more desirable.

How long does treatment take to work?

Any study conducted to determine whether or not a treatment is effective for hair loss lasts at least one year. This does not mean that it takes a whole year to see results. Improvement may be evident as early as 3 months, although 6 months is more realistic. The final results can take a year or more to be fully realized.

There are three clinical indicators that may improve to produce a positive response from treatment. These indicators reflect the following (or some combination of the following) three complaints: (1) **shedding hair**; (2) **thin hair**; and (3) **progressive hair loss**.

Hair shedding is probably the most disturbing symptom and it drives women (and me) crazy. There is something about seeing loose hairs in your hands or the shower drain or the comb/brush that elicits panic (fear of going bald). Also, with the onset of a response to topical medication in particular, there often is a transient increase in shedding called "telogen release" caused by new hair growth which pushes out the increased number of resting hairs that often populate the scalp afflicted by FPHL. I tell patients that this indicates that treatment is working, although it doesn't have to occur or be noticeable to get a good result. If shedding is one of your symptoms of FPHL (and not caused by some other condition), there is usually noticeable decrease in shedding around 3 months. However, shedding is often seen periodically, even with a good response to treatment, and is discussed in more detail in Chapter 6 (Telogen Effluvium).

Hair thinning (i.e., decreased hair volume/mass) takes at least six months to begin to demonstrate improvement using the technique described in Chapter 1. A full response will take a year or more, depending on the hairstyle and length. The studies on men taking Propecia showed gradual improvement in hair density and diameter for up to two years. I tell patients that this is a marathon, not a sprint. It takes patience and endurance to achieve the goal. I see the patient at six-month intervals to monitor their response. Also, when hair volume improves, it occurs from the back toward the front and from the sides toward the midline (part). The area that responds last (and least) is the area in front behind the hairline.

Progressive hair loss is slowed or arrested more predictably than shedding and thinning. Obviously, halting further thinning will not satisfy those patients who have lost so much that there is very noticeable "see through" hair. It also won't (at least initially) satisfy women who started with very thick hair and women who continue to shed more than they consider normal. However, most women notice their loss long before those around them do, and this group will often tell me that they will be very happy if they can just keep the hair they've got. Also, patients who fail to get back their full volume, but improve somewhat, will usually adjust their expectations (if not their desires). Women who are periodic or even persistent "shedders" also learn to appreciate the reality that staying on treatment assures them that their hair will grow back and not continue to become thinner.

How well does treatment work?

In my experience, Female Pattern Hair Loss can be stopped or significantly slowed down in 95% of patients and 60-70% of women may achieve noticeable improvement in hair volume with presently available medical treatments.

As I have discussed previously, my belief is that most women with significant FPHL either do not get adequate treatment or don't take treatment adequately.

But how well does present medical treatment really work for those women I see who are willing to follow my recommendations and "go the distance"?

If there were some dramatic "cure" for everyone with FPHL, I wouldn't need to write this book. So the answer to this very important question is *a priori* nuanced. The criteria for success depend upon the following factors: (1) the **baseline exam**; (2) the patient's **medical condition**; (3) the patient's **expectations/needs**; and (4) the patient's **ability to get and take the medication**.

The best results are achieved in women with less loss and a shorter duration of hair loss. There is no presently available medical treatment that can restore hair in an area where there is none (or only "peach fuzz"). Most women seen in consultation have a graded-rating score (see Chapter 1, Problem #4) of between 2 and 3 in the thinning areas. If there are large numbers of hairs that are visible, but of diminished diameters, there is a reasonable expectation that treatment will result in a noticeable increase in the graded-rating score. If the score increases to 3 or higher, the patient will no longer have that "see-through" look and the treatment can be considered a success if it holds.

Patients with underlying medical conditions, especially endocrine disorders like thyroid imbalances or polycystic ovarian syndrome (see Chapter 7) are less likely to achieve the desired results with present treatment. Also, patients in poor health due to chronic illnesses requiring multiple medications may not be able to use or tolerate the oral medications used for FPHL.

The biggest obstacle in achieving success with present treatment is the underlying psychological and perceptual state of the patient herself. A woman who started with a "crowning glory" (graded-rating score of 5) prior to onset of hair loss may never be satisfied with only modest improvement. A very small group of women, usually in their teens or early 20s, will contentiously contend that they are definitely getting worse despite whatever my objective scores are. I believe that better technology to monitor hair density and volume will still never convince some patients that they are really getting benefits from treatment. They want their original hair fully restored and will not settle for anything less. These patients can sometimes benefit from low dose anti-depressant medications. However, most patients are thrilled and grateful to find a caring physician with helpful treatment and either have or develop realistic expectations and goals. And there is a sizeable group that gets really great results.

Finally, the patient must be able to get and willing to take the treatment. Insurance plans do not have to pay for medications (both topical and systemic) for FPHL since it is not a disease per se. Topical minoxidil (Rogaine) is always an out-of-pocket expense. Many plans exclude medication prescribed off-label, which could apply to all the oral treatments we use. Spironolactone is most likely to succeed for coverage since it is used commonly as a diuretic in both men and women. Finasteride (Propecia/Proscar) and dutasteride (Avodart) are sometimes covered, but I tell patients not to expect it to happen. So treatment can impose a financial burden that not every woman is able to carry. Some women simply draw a line in the sand when it comes to taking something by mouth long term for FPHL. This decision may be philosophical, which

I understand and respect, or because of fear of side effects, which is discussed elsewhere (see below).

How long does treatment go on?

"How long do I have to use this treatment if it works?" asks Tara, age 50.

"Until we get a better treatment or your hair is not important, whichever comes first," responds Dr Reed.

Unfortunately, FPHL doesn't reverse itself and results obtained with present treatment can be expected to be lost gradually if the medication is discontinued. Patients need to know, however, that they will not be worse off for having been on a course of treatment. After some unpredictable time period off therapy, the patient will revert to her "wild state" and look the same, **just as if she were never treated**. Also, FPHL, although usually slowly progressive, may stabilize for long periods of time. There are some patients who may have stabilized prior to starting treatment. If they obtain only slight improvement and stop taking the medication, they may not notice any dramatic decrease in hair volume since the loss would not have progressed much even if they were never treated. Of course, the opposite may also be true. If we have halted ongoing loss that would have been very significant, the poor patient could end up much worse than they might expect.

How lucky do you feel?

Some patients really want to know (if, for some reason, they are uncertain) how helpful the treatment has been. I tell them that they can try taking a break and see what transpires. If there is any significant increase in either shedding or thinning, they should restart the treatment. I have no objections if this is what someone wants to do, but don't wait too long to restart the treatment or it may not be possible to avoid ending up with less hair.

Finally, I tell every patient to get into a one-year time mindset, rather than thinking she will be on treatment the rest of her life. Any study done to determine whether or not a medication can help hair loss is at least one year, sometimes two. Patients may see results as early as 3 months, but I tell them that they must stay with the regimen for one year before making a decision on how well it worked. I see the patient at 6-month intervals. More often visits are usually unhelpful and less frequent visits result in poor patient compliance with attendant poor results. Patients unable or unwilling to develop the mindset needed to "go the distance" are usually lost to follow up soon after the initial consultation. Successful treatment for hair loss is for people who understand the concept of deferred gratification.

Are there any common or serious side effects?

treatment. Sometimes, the problem can be solved by reducing the concentration used (e.g., 6% to 3%). Finally, I have seen a handful of patients who think they notice some slight increase in body hair with higher strength minoxidil, but it is not enough to cause them to stop using it.

Side effects from low-level laser treatment (LLLT) are really minimal. Telogen release was observed in the clinical study, which I interpret as an indication that treatment stimulates hair growth. Minimal local symptoms, like itching, can occur, but I am not aware of any patients who have had to stop treatment due to side effects. Lack of side effects, however, does cause some concern as to how efficacious this kind of treatment is, as discussed at the beginning of this section.

Side effects from systemic therapy have been touched on in the previous section, but require further discussion. However, I am not going to make a laundry list of the information contained in the product package insert. Most women are familiar with potential side effects related to oral contraceptives and hormone replacement therapy. The most common complaints that I get from patients on Yasmin are weight gain, breast sensitivity/enlargement and mood alterations. Spironolactone can also affect the patient's mood in higher doses (200 mg). Some women report an increase in urination (it is a diuretic, albeit a weak one). Occasionally, breast tenderness and menstrual irregularities are seen (usually in higher doses also). Elevated blood potassium (hyperkalemia) is not a problem in healthy women unless (maybe) they are taking excessive potassium supplements as discussed above. Some doctors begin with lower doses of spironolactone (25-50 mg daily) and gradually increase to therapeutic levels (100-200 mg daily) to allow the patient to adjust to and better tolerate the treatment. In my experience the medication least likely to have side effects is finasteride (1 mg or 5 mg). I have seen very few patients who experience either a change in libido or slight breast tenderness. Avodart is more likely to affect libido. I suggest that women take it shortly after sexual activity to ameliorate this problem, if it occurs. For the record, however, I have never had a female patient go off these oral medications because of sexual side effects.

Patients often express concern about problems associated with long-term use of medication. Since treatment for FPHL itself is "long term," this question is understandable. However, there is a general rule that the longer an individual is on a medication, the less likely she will experience adverse reactions. Most of the medications we use for hair loss have been around for many years and we have a good safety profile based on use experience. Even Avodart, the "new kid on the block," has been in use for hair loss since 2002. There is an equilibrium (balance) that is reached between any medication and your body. A drug is absorbed, distributed, metabolized and excreted (pharmacokinetics). It does not "build up in your system." It does what it does to you (pharmacodynamics) and is eliminated from your body. There can never be zero risk, of course. Every time you cross the street, you risk getting hit by a motor vehicle. The same way you can avoid getting run over, you can avoid adverse effects from medication. BE ALERT! If you do not feel well on medication, consult your doctor. Get blood tests, if recommended. Don't miss follow-up visits. If you want zero risk, avoid treatment entirely (and never cross the street!).

Summary

We have made great progress in the treatment for FPHL since I entered this field in 1978. Most patients can look forward to slowing/stopping and, to a lesser degree, reversing their hair loss. Of course, we still have a long way to go before treatment becomes simple and easy. Too many women continue to experience frustration and disappointment with the amount of improvement gained relative to the time, effort and expense involved. But the future is bright (see Chapter 7).

Finally, many women, having controlled and improved their hair loss with medical treatment, still have either a wider part than is desirable or an area right behind the frontal hairline that still has a "see-through" look. These patients are often excellent candidates for the latest techniques for surgical correction that are discussed next in Chapter 5 (What is the surgical treatment for Female Pattern Hair Loss?).

5

WHAT IS THE SURGICAL TREATMENT FOR FEMALE PATTERN HAIR LOSS?

"I have been on the best medical treatment for almost a year and a half. I have stopped losing my hair and noticed definite improvement. However, I still have an area in my frontal scalp that is noticeably thin. What else can I do?" says Elise, age 58.

"A transplant is not an option for me. I heard it is too painful and doesn't work in women," says Celeste, age 47.

"My hair transplant has been a miracle. I can now look in the mirror without fearing that people are going to see my scalp unless I expend a lot of time and effort to disguise the thinned areas. I cannot begin to express my gratitude for what you have done for me," says Roslyn, age 52.

Hair transplantation was discussed briefly in Chapter 1 where my message was that most women should probably get medical treatment first and hold off on surgery until they achieve the full benefits from non-surgical options. However, when the time is right and the female patient is ready, surgical hair replacement can result in some of the happiest and most grateful women ever treated for hair loss.

What is a hair transplant?

A hair transplant is a surgical procedure in which intact, living hair follicles are removed from the back of the head (donor site) and implanted into thinning or balding areas on the crown (recipient site). After an 8-12 week rest period, the hairs begin to grow and can usually be expected to live as long as they would have lived in their original location.

Who should get a transplant?

Any woman who has adequate hair quality/density in the donor region and either has had an inadequate response to medical treatment or whose loss is too far advanced for non-surgical treatment may be a candidate for this procedure.

When do you need a hair transplant?

You may need (i.e., can benefit from) a transplant if you still have a graded-rating density score (see Chapter 1, Problem #4) of 2.5 or less in the area(s) of hair loss after an adequate course of medical treatment (see Chapter 4). Also, if you are seeking treatment for the first time and have an area (usually in the frontal scalp) that has a density score of 2.0 or less, a transplant may be the only way to get noticeable improvement.

How do they do a hair transplant?

There are several variations of the modern day surgical technique called "follicular unit" transplantation. Hairs on the scalp grow in naturally occurring clusters of individual hair follicles surrounded by non-follicular fibrous tissue. In the peripheral areas like the frontal hairline, these units contain 1-2 hairs and in the central regions there are 2-4 hair units. Hairs taken from the donor site are used to restore these missing units using very tiny pieces of scalp (grafts) with one or two follicular units (1-4 hairs) in each graft. The goal is to recreate a pattern and distribution of transplanted hair that is both natural looking and dense.

The most common procedure is called "strip harvesting." A long and narrow section of scalp is excised under local anesthesia. A typical strip is approximately ½ inch wide by 6-8 inches in length and contains 2500-4000 hair follicles. The strip of scalp is then micro dissected into the little hair-containing grafts mentioned above. Micro forceps are used to place these grafts into tiny openings in the recipient areas that are created using a variety of small incision-making devices (needles, blades, punches, etc.). These grafts "stick" in the scalp and form small crusts that heal in 1-2 weeks. Hair regrowth begins generally in 8-12 weeks. Sutures (stitches) used to close the donor site are removed after about 2 weeks. A thin linear scar is left that is covered by the hair above it.

A newer technique called "follicular unit extraction" (FUE) has evolved over the past few years. In this procedure there is no strip excision. Instead, the operator uses a micro punch that is less than 1/25 of an inch in diameter to "extract" individual 1-3 hair follicular units in large numbers under local anesthesia. This procedure is longer and more labor intensive than the strip method and sometimes requires more than one procedure to achieve the desired density. However, it is much less invasive and the healing or "down time" is greatly reduced. There are no sutures, no linear scar, and minimal/absent post-op pain/discomfort.

The strip method is generally preferred for a first time procedure in a patient with a recipient site that is very thin (or bald) and very large. It is the best way to get the most density in the shortest time and with the least effort. Women desire density most of all and this technique can provide it, especially if the grafts contain 3-5 hairs (2-unit grafts) and are put very close together (so-called dense packing). However, if the patient has a smaller area such as the treatment-resistant post-frontal area or a widened part, FUE may be preferable. It can increase the density of any thin hair region and is a much gentler procedure, which is appealing to many female patients.

Both techniques have a place in female hair restoration. In my experience, a lot of women who have been unwilling to undergo a strip excision are likely to undergo an FUE procedure due to the short (4-5 day) down time, minimal discomfort and reduced "shock loss" (see below).

More information on how we perform hair transplantation, including viewing a live surgery, can be obtained on my web site (www.MichaelReedMD.com).

How long does a hair transplant last?

As mentioned above, transplanted hair is expected to live as long in its new home at the recipient site as it would have lived in the donor area. Of course, it must survive the relocation process (transplant). Most experienced surgeons with well-trained tissue-handling technicians can probably boast 95% (or greater) follicular survival.

The problem that arises with female patients is the concern that women are likely to experience gradual thinning over their entire scalp. So it is possible that the transplanted hairs may not last for a lifetime. However, even if this is true, it doesn't preclude performing a transplant and getting great benefits. First, it's not as if the transplanted hairs don't survive. They definitely do. And what if they live for 10 years instead of the rest of the patient's life? That's still a long time. Truthfully, in my 30+ years of experience in transplantation, I can't recall any female patient who ever lost much of their transplanted hair. I think the reason for this is that even though the hair of the donor site may be diminished in volume over a lifetime, it is not "lost." The average hair diameter may decrease, but the hair doesn't stop growing (i.e., become invisible). Also, I think that by the time a woman needs a transplant, her donor site has already finished thinning out and is stable. So the hairs that are transplanted probably will survive a very long time, if not a lifetime.

Does a transplant eliminate the need for other treatments?

The concern that transplanted hair may not survive over time can be ameliorated by keeping the patient on maintenance medical therapy. However, the main reason to continue medical treatment is to prevent further loss of the rest of the non-transplanted hair. Women really don't want to "chase baldness" with a transplant every so many years as their FPHL slowly progresses. Eventually, the donor site becomes depleted and the game is over. There is not enough donor hair to repopulate the potential area of loss on the top of the head. Chasing hair loss with multiple transplants over time is a losing proposition.

Ongoing medical treatment is thus desirable for most patients. Also, I have had patients who, prior to treatment, had donor sites that were inadequate for transplantation. After a year or so, however, the donor hair had thickened up enough to make them a surgical candidate. Obviously, these women need to remain on medical treatment if they want to maintain the best results.

Finally, a number of women, for many reasons, want a transplant and prefer either to stop medical treatment or to not go on it in the first place. Even though FPHL is usually a slowly progressive process, it can slow down or stabilize over time. Women don't usually "go bald." There is some "end point" that cannot be predicted. If a patient has been on treatment for at least one year and there has been no improvement and their hair loss was rather stable for a few years prior to therapy, they may be able to do a transplant and do okay without medication. It's a calculated risk, but if they are monitored at 6-month intervals and alert to watching for hair thinning/shedding, they may be okay for a long time. I have no objection to this approach, if the criteria outlined above are met or if thc patient insists and is willing to accept the potential risk of further loss.

Why don't more women get transplants?

More women should be getting hair transplants. And more are getting transplants than ever before. In 1978 I would almost never perform a transplant on a woman. Today, in my practice, more than half of transplant cases are women. In the big clinic operations the percentage is smaller, but increasing gradually. The reason for this difference is mostly related to how patients find their way to a transplant (see below).

Women are generally more reluctant to undergo surgery than their male counterparts. In fact, a lot of men are more likely to desire surgery than medical intervention. Women are exactly the opposite. This has to do with the potential sexual side effects of oral medication. Men may tolerate invasive surgery more than women, but if you even suggest the possibility of sexual side effects, many guys will "wimp out." Arguments about the "stronger sex" require a context obviously. So now that we have the less invasive FUE procedure, many more women are becoming enthusiastic candidates for transplantation.

What is the most difficult part of a transplant?

The most difficult part of a transplant for women is something called "shock loss." Most women still have noticeable amounts of hair, albeit thinned out, in their recipient site that is "working overtime" so to speak. The transplanted hairs are carefully placed in between these residual native hairs. Great care is taken to avoid damaging these survivors since they are needed to enhance the final density of the procedure. Nevertheless, the trauma to the area from the local anesthetic and myriad tiny incisions usually "shocks" these fragile natives and variable numbers will be precipitated into the resting (telogen) phase. They subsequently are shed and do not begin to regrow until 2-3 months later, which is when the transplanted hairs also "wake up" and make new hair shafts. So the patient usually has **less hair** than before the procedure for 3-4 months after the surgery. About 20% of patients have enough shock loss to create a coiffing challenge for this time period. Different styling, headbands, cosmetic camouflage and, rarely, a small hairpiece (weft) may be needed.

However, the reward of new, long-living, abundant hair regrowth more than makes up for this temporary situation. Finally, even though many patients express concern about this potential problem, most find the degree of loss minimal and quite tolerable.

What are the potential complications from a transplant?

Side effects are uncommon and manageable in most cases. The worst things include post-op infections, usually in the donor region. This is extremely rare if antibiotics are used preventatively. Poor graft survival, in my opinion, is usually the result of poor tissue handling by the surgical team. Ingrown hairs and cysts are common when hair regrowth begins (8-12 weeks). They usually resolve without treatment or can be easily eliminated by opening them or by giving a local cortisone shot.

There are also post-op side effects that are not really side effects, but rather *sequelae*. These are conditions that are simply part of the post-op course. There is a variable amount of pain, primarily at the donor site after the strip procedure. This is expected and easily managed with simple pain medications. Most patients don't need to take the medication for more than 3 days. A small number of individuals report either much less or much more discomfort. I have heard of patients who report persistent pain, but I have never had such a patient and believe that other factors may be at work in such rare cases unrelated to the actual transplant. However, it is very common for these patients to experience residual numbness or tingling at or over the donor site. These funny sensations (dysesthesia) gradually resolve over 6-12 months in the majority of patients. Rarely, they persist longer. However, I have never had a patient who found the sensations problematic. It is also quite common to get swelling of the forehead that can extend down around the eyes several days after a transplant, resulting in a puffy look. This resolves in 3-4 days and, aside from looking funny, has no adverse effect on the results. Shock loss was described above. Little scabs form over the grafts that fall off in 5-14 days.

Some residual pinkish discoloration may persist for some weeks, but is really mild and disappears fairly quickly.

In my opinion, there are no potential side effects (or sequelae) that should prevent a woman from getting a transplant if she needs and desires one.

Where should I go for a transplant?

Hair transplants are performed by a large array of medical specialists besides dermatologists. This is a wide-open field of endeavor. Patients sometimes express concern when they find out their eye doctor or internist has started learning how to perform hair transplantation. As a dermatologist, I confess my bias about where women (and men) should go for this type of procedure. Dermatologists pioneered this field and we also are trained in the diagnosis and treatment of all kinds of hair loss disorders. I see a lot of patients who I talk out of surgery in favor of a medical approach. I believe that the patient has a greater chance of getting what she really needs from a dermatologist, even if she initially thinks she wants just a transplant.

On the other hand, the influx of talented practitioners from other branches of medicine and surgery has contributed greatly to advances in the field. There is no reason why a trained physician can't become an excellent transplant surgeon. In fact, the really valuable individuals in the operating room are probably the non-physician tissue-handling technicians. In larger clinic-type operations, these technicians do the lion's share of the work. And in the latest FUE technique, a non-physician surgical specialist often does even more of the procedure. However, in all cases, the senior surgeon supervises the team and is required to perform the surgical excision of the donor strip.

Women are less inclined to go to a large franchise-type transplant center than men. In my lengthy experience, the female patient prefers to find an individual surgeon with experience and a good reputation. Ideally, she wants to get a referral from someone she trusts, like her own doctor or a knowledgeable close friend or relative. A trusted hair stylist or colorist may be able to provide a referral. Finally, your local dermatologist either should know about or be able to easily find out about good surgeons in your area. Surfing the Internet is more risky in my opinion, but the Internet can be a good source of information.

Free consultations are appealing and may be helpful for some people, but there is an intrinsic risk with them. You are more likely to get a sales pitch and less likely to get professional advice, which is what you really want. If you pay for a consultation, you have a better chance of getting the best counsel since the doctor is compensated for his/her valuable time, effort and expertise. Most surgeons will deduct the consultation fee from the cost of the procedure if it is done within a reasonable time after the visit. Remember the economic dictum: *You don't get what you don't pay for*. On the other hand, you can still be taken advantage of if the surgeon is predatory or mercenary (yes, they exist). Perhaps this is a shocking revelation to a few of my readers. Trust your intuition and life experience. If you don't like the surgeon or feel that something is not right, don't sign up for any procedure. Get other opinions!

Summary

Hair transplantation has come a very long way from the old days of large plug-type procedures. The fact that I can write this chapter for women and recommend the latest techniques with enthusiasm is a testimony to our immense progress in the field. More than half the patients that I perform transplant surgery on today are women, and I expect this percentage to continue increasing because of the newer FUE method and because women tend to seek out physicians like myself who have expertise in both medical and surgical arenas. The number of females treated in large clinic-type practices will also increase, albeit more slowly, because of how women seek professional help.

The present technique of moving large numbers of 1-4 hair follicular units from the back of the head to the top has probably reached its zenith in terms of being safe and effective as I write this book. But there is still room for significant further progress. The donor site is limited and often lacks the density required to give women the full restoration they desire. The procedures are tedious, labor intensive and relatively costly for many women. Potential shock loss is an obstacle for a lot of patients, even though it is rarely as significant as they think it will be. But it would be really great to further reduce or eliminate their concerns of post-op downtime.

Chapter 7 will briefly discuss what I believe is a bright future for both the medical and surgical approaches to the treatment of FPHL.

6

WHAT IS THE RELATIONSHIP BETWEEN FPHL AND TELOGEN EFFLUVIUM?

"I started treatment for my hair loss about three weeks ago. Now I am losing ***more*** *hair than before! What's going on here?" says Lillian, age 44.*

"I have been on your full treatment for hair loss for a little over one year and was doing really well until two weeks ago when I started to shed hair again. Has the treatment stopped working?" asks Gina, age 37.

"For two years I used the special topical minoxidil and it really worked, so I stopped using it a month ago. Now I'm shedding like crazy even though I restarted it two weeks ago," says Paula, age 53.

"My hair keeps falling out in clumps even though I am doing ***everything right****. All my blood tests are normal. I know there*

is something wrong with me, but no one seems to be able to figure it out. I'm going to end up ***bald*** *at this rate," says Mimi, age 28.*

There is nothing more distressing for a woman with hair loss than seeing loose hairs in the brush or shower drain. I get more calls for this complaint than anything else in my practice. Even when the patient knows what is going on, there is still the uncontrollable fear of going bald.

In my opinion, the condition commonly called Telogen Effluvium (TE) has been taught in a very oversimplified manner to most dermatologists trained to diagnose and treat hair loss disorders. Most textbooks make it sound like an easy (and obvious) diagnosis with a simple treatment (i.e., do nothing).

Textbook (simple/easy) cases of TE probably are rather mild and don't make their way to the dermatologist since they resolve quickly and require no treatment. When I see women who complain about excessive shedding, there is often a complex relationship, sometimes involving underlying systemic conditions and frequently overlapping with other common hair loss disorders like female pattern hair loss (FPHL) and alopecia areata (see Chapter 7).

Cases of Telogen Effluvium (TE) seen in my office are usually complex and treatment is often problematic. Simple TE, as described in dermatology textbooks, is usually only found in the textbooks! Read on.

What exactly is Telogen Effluvium?

Telogen Effluvium is an increased loss of normal resting (telogen) hair shafts with the characteristic little white follicular root/bulb. These are also called "club" hairs. It is normal for about 5% of scalp hairs to be in the resting phase of the hair growth cycle, and these are the hairs that come out when we wash or comb our hair. A typical person will shed 30-50 hairs daily, maybe up to 100 depending upon how often hair washing occurs. However, whether you wash daily or weekly, the average remains the same. Women experiencing a shedding period will invariably decrease their washing frequency. Understandably, you don't like to see your hair coming out in the shower. Of course, this only postpones the distress, since even larger numbers of hair will come out when you do wash. Plus, you may be walking around with greasy hair that doesn't look very nice, right?

Something happens in the body that "shocks" a large number of your growing hair follicles so that they prematurely go into the resting phase. These resting (telogen) hairs are not anchored deeply like growing (anagen) hairs and come out more easily with normal manipulation during washing and styling. The resting period is usually 3-4 months before a new hair starts to grow, pushing out these telogen hairs. The new hair then has to grow to a certain length to provide coverage. Scalp hair typically grows about one-half inch a month. The number of resting hairs in TE is quite variable, but in more severe cases can be up to 50%.

Simple cases of so-called acute telogen effluvium occur after a number of different circumstances. This is when there is a finite event/insult such as a febrile illness (an illness with a fever) or sudden weight loss. These women may not connect the precipitating cause with the shedding due to the 2-4 month hiatus. However, most of the time the shedding is either relatively mild or fairly brief and medical help is not sought out. These women are almost never seen for a hair loss consultation. They don't need one.

So let's talk about those patients who shed hair and need my expertise.

Who gets Telogen Effluvium?

Women are shedders. It is unusual to see men for male pattern hair loss (MPHL) that is manifested by excessive falling hair. An overwhelming number of female pattern hair loss (FPHL) patients present with shedding as one of several hair loss symptoms (discussed in Chapter 2). Shedding is invariably associated with thinning, of course. For years I have tried to ask every new patient whether shedding or thinning came first. Most of the time they are unable to answer this question. The ostensible reason for obtaining this historical information is to determine if the patient has telogen effluvium (TE) or FPHL. The sudden onset of large amounts of loose hairs is typical for acute TE. Gradually thinning hair over time is fairly typical for FPHL. But a lot of patients with FPHL have persistent shedding, albeit less than TE, along with thinning. Women with

FPHL, in my experience, are also more prone to TE. Finally, significant shedding in a short time frame can cause some noticeable thinning with TE. This overlap muddies the water in many cases.

The lucky women with straightforward acute TE have an identifiable precipitating cause or event 2-4 months prior to a rather abrupt onset of shedding. In my practice, the most common causes include going on/off oral contraceptives, rapid and/or significant weight loss and surgical procedures with general anesthesia. Shedding after pregnancy (post-partum TE) is quite common, but generally not severe or persistent enough to see a hair loss specialist.

Hair loss associated with oral medications is sometimes difficult to diagnose. It seems that most package inserts report a 1-2% incidence of drug-related hair loss. This kind of information is not very helpful. I believe it is more useful to determine the time frame relationship if a medication is suspected. If shedding starts within a period of several weeks or months after starting a new medication, it should be suspect. There are, of course, a number of medications that are known to induce hair loss. I am not going to attempt to provide an exhaustive list here. However, the types of drug categories that I have seen most commonly include medications used for high blood pressure, high cholesterol, neurochemical imbalances and blood thinners. The only way to know if your new medication is causing your hair loss is to stop it (if medically safe to do so) and see if your shedding stops and your hair recovers, which can, unfortunately, take 6-12 months. Ideally, you should also restart the drug and see if your loss recurs. Of course, no one wants to do this unless they absolutely have to for medical reasons. I also believe that in many patients, the body adjusts to a new medication and the hair loss abates without having to stop treatment. Often, fortunately, there may be safer alternative drugs available if it is fairly certain that a medication is causing ongoing loss.

How do you diagnose Telogen Effluvium (TE)?

The diagnosis of TE is usually made based upon a history of a rather abrupt onset of excessive shedding compared to the patient's usual observations of loose hairs in the comb/brush and/or shower drain. The loose hairs usually have a tiny white bulb at the end. As discussed above, there should be some precipitating cause 2-4 months prior to onset.

If there is any doubt about the diagnosis, we can send a sample of loose hairs to the dermatopathology lab for a trichogram (hair examination under the light microscope) to confirm that there is no hair shaft or hair root disorder (see Chapter 7). In addition, the patient can do a loose hair collection and count (see Chapter 1, Problem #5). Normally, the average daily shed is under 50 hairs. Up to 100 hairs is said to be normal in textbooks, but I think that is rather on the high side. Patients with TE can have peak shedding days of over 300 hairs and rarely even higher. The time from start to finish for an episode of TE is variable, but usually occurs in a 2-4 month time frame. However, it will take about a year for hair volume to recover.

Are there different types of Telogen Effluvium?

Yes and no. We usually say that there are two varieties of TE based upon the duration of the shedding period: **ACUTE TE** or **CHRONIC TE**. This is oversimplified to the point of being a bit misleading. Sometimes a typical case of textbook-type acute TE can persist well beyond a 2-4 month period (i.e., become chronic TE). Other times, chronic TE comes and goes like recurring episodes of acute TE, but without any identifiable causes.

How confusing is this? I shall try to shed some light on these observations below when I discuss the relationship between TE and FPHL.

There are also several types of treatment-related TE that are rather common, much to the chagrin of both the patient and me. Following is a list of these types of shedding with my interpretation of what is going on with each:

1. **Telogen Release** – When you start treatment for FPHL, you may have a large number of hairs in the resting phase. The treatment will cause these hairs to go into the growing phase over a period of several weeks to months. These resting hairs are "pushed out" by the new growth. The amount of shedding is usually rather mild, but may not be perceived that way by an anxious patient who is focused on her hair. Even though I tell every patient about this potential phenomenon, we get more calls about telogen release than almost anything else. The worst thing to do, of course, is to stop the treatment just as it is beginning to work. Telogen

release seems to be associated mostly with initiation of topical minoxidil. It is very unusual, however, for the amount of shedding to cause any noticeable hair thinning unless a patient has extremely thin areas to begin with.

2. **Synchronized Shedding** – Humans don't usually shed like other animals since all our scalp hairs are in individual hair cycles so that only a small percentage shed at the same time. However, when you start treatment for hair loss, you may initiate new growth for a large number of hairs at the same time. Eventually, these "synchronized" hairs may rest, and then shed around the same time. It is common for this phenomenon to occur toward the end of the first and second years of treatment, often being most noticeable in the fall or spring, depending on when you started your treatment. In a typical case the patient reports that, after improving or stabilizing for a number of months, they are rather suddenly shedding like before or at the beginning of treatment. They wonder if the treatment has stopped working. Again I say that this is not the case at all and not to stop treatment. In fact, I say that the treatment is their best assurance that the hairs will grow back.[1]

---

1 I have observed that when patients stay on treatment for three or more years, these periods of shedding seem to diminish, probably because gradually the individual hair cycles become asynchronous again. I think it is interesting that clinical studies lasting 1-2 years may conclude that the test medication loses some efficacy. This may not be true since measurements of hair density will decrease after episodes of synchronized shedding. So be careful if you read somewhere that medications like minoxidil gradually become ineffective. That has not been my experience over time.

3. **Idiopathic Shedding** – There are many times when, despite performing the "million dollar" work-up, no cause can be found for episodes of shedding. Fortunately, these shedding periods are usually self-limited and do not result in noticeable hair thinning in a majority of women.

4. **Seasonal Shedding** – It is common for people to experience an increase in hair shedding in the fall season and, to a lesser degree, in the springtime. When women have hair loss and go on treatment, they may be more likely to notice shedding because of heightened awareness and call to report it.

What is the relationship between Telogen Effluvium (TE) and Female Pattern Hair Loss (FPHL)?

First, let me point out the differences since these are two different kinds of hair loss. The main feature of FPHL that is supposed to be absent in all of the above variations of TE is the process of hair follicle (and thus also hair shaft diameter) miniaturization (shrinkage). Also, the degree and duration of shedding is different, although in both cases the shed hairs are normal telogen hairs. Acute TE as described above is easy to tell apart from FPHL. Chronic TE of undetermined cause is more difficult since both disorders have persistent shedding and decreased scalp hair. However, the shedding associated with chronic TE tends to have more dramatic ups and downs and may have periods of remission that are sometimes predictable. The main feature of chronic TE is lack of hair miniaturization. If it is difficult to determine this finding with a scalp exam, I will send a sampling of loose hairs to the lab to measure hair diameters.

But now things start to get more complicated. Over time many patients with recurrent or persistent TE will develop FPHL. I believe that in most cases these individuals were genetically predisposed to FPHL and it has been "unmasked" somewhat prematurely by whatever incident(s) caused episodes of TE. A common example is multiple pregnancies. After the first child, an episode of TE resolves and the hair volume is restored. But with successive children, there is less recovery and at some point the diagnosis of FPHL is established (unless, of course, the joys of raising multiple children results in excessive hair pulling!).

Could chronic TE really be a form of FPHL in which the sensitivity to androgens is manifested as a shortened growing time without the usual shrinkage of the follicle seen in FPHL? Many cases of chronic TE seem to be associated with underlying thyroid problems. However, adequate treatment of the thyroid condition(s) may not have a beneficial effect on the persistent hair shedding. Thyroid hormones have a role in the hair growth cycle, and untreated thyroid problems are characterized by changes in hair growth and texture. Is there some kind of problem with the interaction of thyroid hormone with the hair follicle that adversely affects the hair growth cycle? We don't know.

One thing is quite certain, however. And that is the observation that a majority of women who come for a consultation for hair loss associated with excessive shedding have underlying diagnosable FPHL with or without a form of TE. Remember that these are the two most common kinds of hair loss, and so it is expected that they might overlap, even if they were totally different in every other way. However, as I have stated previously, I believe that women with FPHL have hair that is more susceptible to events/conditions that result in TE. So I view them as traveling companions.

When TE and FPHL occur together, there is often confusion about which condition is dominant and what should be the approach to treatment. Treatment for FPHL has been discussed in Chapter 4. What about TE? Read on.

How do you treat Telogen Effluvium?

As stated previously, no treatment is needed for simple acute TE that doesn't have an underlying condition such as FPHL. But how do you know whether or not you have an underlying tendency for FPHL that may be revealed by acute TE?

I think we have to try a common sense approach here, even though the answer to the above question is: **you don't know**!

What if you have a very strong family history of hereditary MPHL/FPHL, a history of episodic hair loss (that recovered) and your shedding is really severe? In this scenario, it might be worth getting treatment to cover you for the possibility of an incomplete recovery due to unmasking a tendency for underlying FPHL. You could get treatment for

FPHL and try stopping it in 6-12 months when your TE finished its course. The decision is like gambling based on uncertain probabilities. How lucky are you? Should you gamble with your hair?

It's your call.

There is no guaranteed treatment for idiopathic (i.e., unknown cause) episodic or chronic TE. Undiagnosed underlying conditions discovered by the blood testing suggested in Chapter 1 may be detected, but usually everything is normal in the woman who is healthy except for her hair loss. I do find a lot of women with low normal blood ferritin levels. There is some study data suggesting that you should keep your blood ferritin (body iron storage protein) level above 50 ng/ml if you have hair loss, especially if you are a shedder. Topical minoxidil can help you recover a little more quickly from acute TE, but is less helpful with chronic TE.

I think there are several hypothetical kinds of TE that may exist, but we don't have objective tests yet to prove (or disprove) their existence. The only "proof," if I dare call it that, is based on anecdotal clinical experience. I call the two "conditions" (1) **Inflammatory** TE and (2) **Neurogenic** TE. It is known that patients who have persistent shedding of undetermined cause may sometimes respond to an intramuscular shot of cortisone. I have had patients report a rather sudden decrease in shedding after such treatment. In these individuals, some local or systemic inflammatory (possibly allergic) factors may be operating. In other patients I have seen hair shedding associated with noticeable and disturbing burning sensations of the scalp. These individuals may respond to low dose SSRI (selective serotonin release-uptake inhibitors) medications. However, remember that sometimes these commonly prescribed anti-depressants may actually worsen loss. They may also work indirectly to reduce to psychological suffering associated with hair loss. I have used them with success in selected patients. I know for a fact that the treatment helps ameliorate the abnormal scalp sensations. However, most patients with increased scalp sensitivity and FPHL have an increase in the androgen content of their hair follicles, which can cause similar, albeit less severe, symptoms. So neurogenic TE might simply be a variant of FPHL associated with excess shedding. Hypothetically, neurogenic hair loss could be caused by some abnormal activity in the nerve fibers that surround the hair follicle. This activity is presumably a neurochemical that directly or indirectly causes the hair to go into the telogen (resting) phase.

Summary

There is nothing more disturbing for the patient and more frustrating for the doctor than the extra hair shedding associated with both an underlying hair loss disorder (FPHL) and a treatment-related event (e.g., synchronized shedding, seasonal shedding, etc.). The good news is that if you stay with the treatment program, your condition is very unlikely to deteriorate over time, assuming you cover yourself for the possibility of underlying FPHL. And, if you just have chronic TE, you will never go bald because the hair will always grow back. From time to time, those loose hairs that come and go in the shower may still bother you. However, once you know your own individual times and circumstances of shedding, you will be much less disturbed by the fear of going bald.

7

WHAT ABOUT ALL THE OTHER KINDS OF HAIR LOSS DISORDERS?

"I know that I have Female Pattern Hair Loss, but is it possible that something else is going on here?" asks Emily, age 32.

"Shouldn't I get blood tests to find out the cause of my hair loss?" asks Angela, age 45.

"My stylist found a bald spot on the back of my head and told me I might go bald. Is it true?" asks Melanie, age 23.

This book is written primarily for women afflicted with Female Pattern Hair Loss and her "little sister" Telogen Effluvium. However, there are several other kinds of hair loss that are also fairly common and a much longer list of uncommon or rare disorders. In addition, there are some scalp conditions such as psoriasis and seborrheic dermatitis that are very common and often travel along with FPHL and other hair loss disorders. Here is where your local dermatologist is capable of treating you so you don't have to find a hair loss specialist.

It is beyond the purpose and scope of this book to go into great depth about other kinds of hair loss. That might be material for a sequel. However, I shall try to outline the most significant conditions and explain how to differentiate them from FPHL, along with some simple treatment advice.

These hair loss disorders will be presented in order of decreasing likelihood.

Do you have alopecia areata?

Alopecia areata is the third most common cause of hair loss, affecting about 2% of the population at one time or another. It is characterized in most cases by one or more totally bald spots of variable size anywhere on the scalp (or body). A lot of people refer to it simply as "alopecia," which is actually incorrect since alopecia just means "hair loss" of any type. More severe involvement can cause total loss of scalp hair (alopecia totalis) or body hair (alopecia universalis).

Most cases are easy to distinguish from FPHL. Sometimes, when patients have diffuse thinning over their entire scalp, there may be a question as to whether the condition is an extensive case of FPHL (alopecia diffusa) versus so-called "diffuse" alopecia areata. However, even in these circumstances, the alopecia areata patient has a noticeable "patchy" pattern that precedes and overlaps with the diffuse loss. In these cases, the hair pull test yields 10+ loose hairs. If there is any doubt, a trichogram may show abnormal (dystrophic) anagen roots. A scalp biopsy, done in an active area of loss may also be diagnostic, but not always. But it is occasionally needed to confirm the diagnosis.

Your local dermatologist has been trained to diagnose and treat alopecia areata. Many, if not most, of these patients will experience spontaneous recovery without any treatment. If the condition is persistent or severe, a dermatologist can prescribe a variety of topical medications or give cortisone shots safely into the affected areas. In more severe cases, it may be necessary to see a hair loss specialist for more complicated local or even systemic therapy.

Do you have a systemic disorder associated with FPHL?

It is very uncommon for a woman with FPHL to have any significant underlying systemic condition lurking in her body, where there are no clues from the history or physical exam suggesting otherwise. Most of the women with underlying systemic disorders already have a diagnosis of the condition prior to seeing me. They come in because treatment for that condition has not helped their hair.

So what should you do if you are reading this book and have hair loss, presumably FPHL, and want to know if something else is going on?

Well, start with other historical/physical findings that may indicate an underlying disorder.

Do you have symptoms of weight gain, irregular menses, persistent acne, unwanted facial/body hair, chronic fatigue, and/or heat or cold intolerance? I know that many of these findings are common in women without hair loss and may be unrelated to systemic disorders. However, if you have multiple conditions that are persistent, severe and in combination with your hair loss, they may indicate that there is some associated hormonal, metabolic or immunologic disorder playing a role in your hair loss.

Further evaluation is needed in these circumstances. We might begin with the blood tests outlined in Chapter 1. However, in cases where these symptoms are multiple and rather severe, it may be more desirable to go straight to an endocrinologist for a more thorough work-up. Most of these patients will discover a problem with their ovaries (e.g., polycystic ovarian syndrome) or their thyroid gland (e.g., Hashimoto's thyroiditis). Insulin-resistant diabetes is fairly common also, particularly in obese individuals. Less common findings include pituitary gland disorders (e.g., prolactinomas) and adrenal gland problems (e.g., adrenal hyperplasia).

In my experience, many of these patients need help from both the endocrinologist **and** the dermatologist for their hair loss. This is probably because the systemic problem unmasks and accelerates an underlying predisposition for FPHL. That's why I tell patients that they should be happy when their blood tests are normal. Underlying conditions make treatment more complicated and problematic in most cases.

In any event, if you have a suspicion that you may have a systemic disorder based upon the presence of the symptoms described above, and have not yet had any blood tests performed, I suggest consulting with an endocrinologist before seeing someone like me. If you are fortunate, you may not need my help.

Do you have Traction Alopecia or Follicular Degeneration Syndrome (FDS)?

Hair loss caused over time by chemical and mechanical insults that result from attempts to control spiral/helical/curly hair texture can eventually result in permanent, irreversible hair loss. This is very common in African-American women who want long hair but have uncooperative hair texture. There is a big overlap here with FPHL. It is interesting that two of the most common patterns of loss are in the fronto-temporal regions and the vertex (central centrifugal cicatricial alopecia). This may correspond to areas of maximal chronic trauma over time but also overlaps with areas affected by androgenic alopecia (androgen-driven hair loss). I think that women with underlying FPHL may be more susceptible to damage caused by application of heat (hot combs), chemicals (relaxers) and tight styling techniques (corn rowing/braiding).

Damage to the permanent upper portion of the hair follicle (called the isthmus) eventually destroys this region and the follicle is replaced by scar tissue. Game over. The term Follicular Degeneration Syndrome (FDS) has generally been used as another term for Traction (or "hot comb") Alopecia. However, there are occasional cases of FDS without any history of chemical/mechanical hair trauma. In my opinion, these cases represent an inflammatory and destructive form of androgenetic alopecia (MPHL/FPHL).

Treatment is primarily directed at minimizing further insults, even if it means keeping a short hairstyle and using wigs for long hair. If underlying FPHL is suspected, it is desirable to use the topical or oral medications discussed in Chapter 3. If there is evidence of scalp irritation, cortisone lotions or local shots can be helpful. If there is permanent hair loss, surgical treatment (transplantation) may be the only way to get more hair. Unfortunately, many older women with traction alopecia have also lost much of the hair in their potential donor region, which limits the potential for surgery.

Do you have some type of scarring alopecia?

The two most common conditions we see in this category are called Lichen Planopilaris (LPP) and Discoid Lupus Erythematosis (DLE). Like traction alopecia, the hair follicles are gradually destroyed. It is not likely that you would confuse these rather uncommon, but not rare, conditions with FPHL. They usually are characterized by either localized or widespread patchy hair loss and are sometimes hard to tell from alopecia areata, unless you are a hair loss specialist. This is a type of hair loss where the scalp biopsy is not only useful for diagnosis, but also for choice of treatment. The biopsy should be taken from the edge of an involved area since that is where the inflammation is active and the findings most likely to result in a correct diagnosis. A biopsy from the center of a bald spot will just show that there is permanent hair follicle destruction, but not diagnose the cause.

There is a form of LPP that is often confused with male pattern hair loss (MPHL) called frontal fibrosing alopecia (FFA). This can be a tricky diagnosis to make, even for your local dermatologist. The inflammatory process involves the peripheral scalp with slow advancement, creating a hat or headband pattern of thinning or absent hairs. Most of the time, the loss is confined to the frontal hairline, but sometimes can spread to the sides and back of the scalp. In the former case, it is often confused with MPHL. In the latter situation, it may look like alopecia areata. There may be visible inflammation manifested as redness at the base of surviving hairs, but not always. However, the involved scalp has a smooth, shiny porcelain-like texture. Close-up examination (dermoscopy) reveals no tiny follicular ostia (pores) seen in MPHL and alopecia areata. You won't be able to see these surface markings easily with the naked eye. That's why we have hair loss specialists.

Treatment for scarring alopecias is complicated and the results unpredictable. The goal is to control the inflammation until the condition burns itself out, usually over several years, but not always. It's like fighting a forest fire to prevent destruction of the trees by containing the fire until the weather changes (i.e., it rains). The latest research indicates that the problem may actually reside in the sebaceous glands due to a malfunction of a receptor (PPAR-gamma) inside the cell nucleus that results in the release of toxic fatty acids which cause an inflammatory reaction that destroys follicles. A drug called Actos™ used in type 2 diabetes is reported to normalize sebaceous gland functions and may become the preferred treatment in the near future. Time will tell. A good local dermatologist may be able to treat milder case with local anti-inflammatory medication (e.g., cortisone) or certain antibiotics. More difficult cases should be sent to a specialist. At a recent dermatology conference, I heard a talk on this subject by a well-known hair loss specialist who works in an academic referral-type practice. He said that fully one third of his patients suffer from these disorders. In my community-based practice, I have many of these patients also, but FPHL/TE cases predominate.

Do you have a hair breakage disorder?

There are a large number of hair shaft disorders that result in unusual hair texture or fragility (breakage). Most of these disorders are uncommon or rare and would not be confused with FPHL. However, it is a fairly common complaint among women with FPHL that their hair texture had changed in some way. It often becomes finer, and less often, frizzier. A lot of patients feel that there is some breakage going on, along with all the other symptoms (see Chapter 2).

Hair breakage disorders are uncommon in women who don't over process their hair with mechanical/thermal/chemical insults. Hair is pretty tough. Of course, as hair lengthens, it "weathers" just like any other non-living tissue (like your clothing). So it is common to see "split ends" (trichoptilosis) in longer haired individuals.

Patients with hair shaft breakage will present complaining that their hair "doesn't grow" rather than it is shedding or thinning. The scalp exam reveals hairs of multiple different lengths. The diagnosis is confirmed by sending loose or clipped hair shafts to the lab for a trichogram. The overwhelming majority of breakage cases are caused by a condition called Trichorrhexis Nodosa. At intervals along the hair shaft there are small "nodes" (bumps). Closer exam of these nodes shows a split with longitudinal fissures. When the hair breaks at this node (called trichoclasis), the end of the hair looks like a small paintbrush.

Gentle hair care, shorter hair styling, special hair care products to strengthen hair and nutritional supplements (see Chapter 3) may be useful. If you also have FPHL, topical minoxidil may be helpful.

Do you have short anagen syndrome?

Short anagen syndrome is supposed to be a rare disorder in which there is a progressive decrease in the duration of the hair growth phase (anagen) so that the hair gets progressively shorter over time.

I have never seen (or been able to diagnose) a case. So I'm not convinced it really exists. The hair shafts and roots are normal if you do a trichogram.

This is a condition to consider if a patient has hair that won't grow and there is no other explanation. It is necessary also to prove that the hair really doesn't grow by shaving or dyeing a clump of hair and watching it over time to confirm the patient's complaint. I saw one patient with this complaint, but he disappeared when I wanted to do this confirmatory test.

Do you have loose anagen syndrome?

Here is another rare condition that would result in an increase in shedding similar to some cases of FPHL (mild shedding) or telogen effluvium (more severe shedding). It's supposed to be seen in young blond women of Scandinavian background. I have seen one case since this book was written. A mother noticed her 9-year-old blond-haired daughter was shedding more hair than usual. She saw several doctors who said there was nothing wrong. However, a loose hair trichogram revealed many anagen hairs with a so-called "ruffled cuticle" that is probably a diagnostic finding for this condition. Fortunately, there is no noticeable thinning and her mother is no longer afraid her daughter will go bald.

Don't expect this diagnosis unless you think all those dumb blond jokes are really true (they're not). There isn't any specific treatment either, but the condition is supposedly mild and gradually diminishes over time.

Do you have trichotillomania?

Lots of women (and men) have a nervous habit of touching their hair. Trichotillomania (TTM) means tricho (hair) tillo (touch) mania (uncontrollable habit). It's not likely that anyone would confuse FPHL with TTM. The serious cases that involve actually pulling out or breaking off of the hair, are usually seen in teenage girls, most of whom deny self-inflicted damage. Sometimes the pattern of hair loss is rather bizarre with short spiky hairs of different lengths on the crown and long silky hairs on the sides of the scalp. At other times there are patchy areas of loss that are often misdiagnosed as alopecia areata. The diagnosis can be confirmed with a scalp biopsy that shows characteristic shattered hair shafts with areas of micro hemorrhaging (bleeding). Treatment involves a combination of individual and family therapy and a good neuropharmacologist.

Do you have Tinea Capitis?

Tinea capitis is a fungal infection that causes one or more patches of hair loss/breakage associated with variable degrees of inflammation (redness, scaling, crusting, etc.). Have you been roughing it in some exotic location recently? Have you picked up a new stray pet that sleeps on your bed? Then maybe you have tinea (fungus) capitis (of the scalp). Most cases seen nowadays in this country are seen in immigrant populations from Africa or Asia.

The diagnosis is made from sending hair pluck samples to the lab for microscopic exam and/or culture. However, keep in mind that most itchy/scaly scalps are caused by either seborrheic dermatitis or psoriasis. Women with FPHL are no more prone to fungus infections than anyone else.

Tinea capitis was rather common a half-century ago. The advent of the oral medication Griseofulvin pretty much eradicated this disorder. We now have several new oral medications that rapidly eliminate this problem.

Summary

Female Pattern Hair Loss is so common that we must always be alert to the possibility of another hair loss disorder being present that is unrelated to FPHL. A lot of people have co-existing seborrheic dermatitis (inflammatory dandruff). This disorder can manifest itself as simple dandruff. In more severe cases, symptoms include itching, burning, redness, and/or crusting that may be localized, patchy or diffuse in its distribution. Also, the same androgens that contribute to hair loss increase scalp sensitivity and increase sebaceous (oil) gland activity (seborrhea) that, in turn, gives rise to inflammation (dermatitis).

It's very likely that your local dermatologist can be helpful to you if have one of these other kinds of hair loss disorders. But you have to make sure that you and your doctor are on the same page here. If you have FPHL and some other problem, it is likely that you may get treatment for that disorder, but not for your co-existing FPHL. Make sure that your doctor tells you **ALL** the diagnoses that are affecting your hair and scalp. And make sure you know what the specific treatment is for each diagnosis. Don't go in for hair loss and just get an anti-dandruff shampoo.

So we have finished our journey with YOU, the reader, as a woman seeking help and hope for your hair loss. My main purpose has been to help you find out how you can get help and realize that there is hope here and now for you. This is a book about fact (today), not fiction (tomorrow).

However, the future for treating FPHL is brighter than ever. In the medical arena, a new group of topical agents called prostaglandin analogues, which may actually convert those "invisible" vellous hairs back into mature visible ones, may become available in the near future. There is already a prostaglandin product on the market that thickens and lengthens eyelashes. In the surgical realm, we may soon be able to create new hair follicles (so-called Follicular Neogenesis) by injecting large numbers of cloned hair stem cells into areas of balding scalp. But don't wait for these newer treatments if you suffer TODAY. I believe that the women who will get the best results with tomorrow's technology will be those who are getting treatment NOW.

ACKNOWLEDGMENTS

The Jewish people – They taught me that if you know something that's worth remembering and you want it to last, **write it down.**

Mark Podwal, M.D. – My friend and esteemed colleague, who created the artwork that was used for the book cover.

Alice Martell – My agent, who worked tirelessly to convince publishers that this book is needed for women with hair loss.

Philip Felig, M.D. – The great endocrinologist, who has been an invaluable help for my patients with systemic disorders that contribute to hair loss.

Jerry Shupack, M.D. – The world's smartest and wisest dermatologist, who was my early mentor and now has become my good friend.

Nancy Schadt – For her good work as my medical illustrator over the years, including the illustration that is in this book.

Bernie Ackerman, M.D. (deceased) – He was a larger than life character who taught me not just dermatopathology, but, as a clinician, how to interpret the interpretation of the dermatopathologist.

Jackie and John Cascarano – My daughter and son-in-law, who stayed on my case to finish this book, and who are helping to get it to the women who need it.

All my women patients with FPHL – For teaching me how to really listen, and learn from them how to write a book that can give them and others help and hope.

REFERENCES

Introduction

Clinton H. "Pay attention to your hair, because everyone else will." www.Hillaryhub.com. Accessed 2007.

Isaiah 3:16-17 in: The Bible. New International Version.

Judges 16:25-30 in: The Bible. New International Version.

Ausubel N. *Jewish Book of Knowledge*. 1964. p. 191, p. 401. 1964.

Heidelberg Catechism 1559.

The Qur'an. Ahmadiyyah Anjuman Isha'at Islan Lahore, Inc. U.S.A. 1995. Chapter 24, Section 4, verse 31 with commentary. p. 685

National Archives & Records Administration photograph. Smith. Item 111-sc-193785. French civilians shave a woman's head as punishment for collaborating with the Germans. 8/29/44.

MSNBC Radio. "Imus in the morning." 4/4/07.

Safire W. "Haircut." *The New York Times*. 1/11/09.

Chapter One

Hillmann K, Blume-Peytavi U. Diagnosis of hair disorders. *Semin Cutan Med Surg* 2009; 28:33-38.

Cohen B. The Cross-Section Trichometer: A new device for measuring hair quantity, hair Loss, and hair growth. *Dermatol Surg* 2008; 34:900-911.

Chapter Two

Price V. Treatment of hair loss. *N Engl J Med* 1999; 341(13):964-973.

The Forbes Consulting Group. Understanding consumer dynamics in the women's thinning hair/hair loss marketplace: A quantitative assessment. December 1999.

Camacho-Martinez FM. Hair loss in women. *Semin Cutan Med Surg* 2009; 22:19-32.

Shapiro J. Hair loss in women. *N Engl J Med* 2007; 357:1620-30.

Olsen EA. Female pattern hair loss. *J Am Acad Dermatol* 2001; 45:S70-S80.

Hillmer AM et al. Susceptibility variants for male pattern baldness on chromosome 20p11. *Nat Genet* 2008; 40:1279.

Richards JB et al. Male pattern baldness susceptibility locus at 20p11. *Nat Genet* 2008; 40:1282.

Marliani Andrea. Does Female Androgenetic Alopecia Really Exist? Or… Low Estrone Alopecia? Alopecia Caused By Insufficient Local Follicular Esrone Activity. International Society of Hair Restoration Surgery 18th Annual Scientific Meeting 2010.

Chapter Three

Trost LB et al. The diagnosis and treatment of iron deficiency and its potential relationship to hair loss. *J Am Acad Dermatol* 2006; 54:824-42.

Colombo VE et al. Treatment of brittle fingernails and onychoschizia with biotin: scanning electron microscopy. *J Am Acad Dermatol* 1990; 23:1127-32.

Kantor J et al. Decreased serum ferritin is associated with alopecia in women. *J Invest Dermatol* 2003; 121:985-988.

Prager N et al. A randomized double blind, placebo-controlled trial to determine the effectiveness of botanically derived inhibitors of 5-alpha-reductase in the treatment of androgenetic alopecia. *J Altern Complement Med* 2002; 8:143-152.

Problems with dietary supplements. *The Medical Letter* 2002; 44 (1140):83. 9/30/02.

Lowenstein EJ. Diagnosis and management of the dermatologic manifestation of the polycystic ovary syndrome. *Dermatol Therapy* 2006; 19:210-223.

Pandit S. et al. Effect of cuscuta reflexa roxb on androgen-induced alopecia. *J Cosm Derm* 2008; 7:199-204.

Chapter Four

Sackett DL et al. Evidence based medicine: what it is and what it isn't: It's about integrating individual clinical experience and the best external evidence. *BMJ* 1996; 312(7023):71-72.

Shapiro J. Safety of topical minoxidil solution: a one-year, prospective observational study. *J Cut Med Surg* 2003; 7:322-29.

Lucky AW et al. A randomized, placebo-controlled trial of 5% and 2% topical minoxidil solutions in the treatment of female pattern hair loss. *J Am Acad Dermatol* 2004; 50:541-543

Satino JL, Markou M. Hair regrowth and increased hair tensile strength using the HairMax LaserComb for low-level laser therapy. *International J of Cosmetic Surgery and Aesthetic Dermatology* 2003; 5(2):113-117.

Pierard-Franchimont C et al. Ketoconazole shampoo: effect of long-term use in androgenetic alopecia. *Dermatology* 1998; 196:474-477.

Jiang J et al. Topical application of ketoconazole stimulates hair growth in C3H/HeN mice. *J Dermatol* 2005; 32:243-247.

Price VH et al. Lack of efficacy of finasteride in postmenopausal women with androgenetic alopecia. *J Am Acad Dermatol* 2000; 43:768-776.

Iorizzo M et al. Finasteride treatment of female pattern hair loss. *Arch Derm* 2006; 142:298-302.

Olsen EA et al. Evaluation and treatment of male and female pattern hair loss. *J Am Acad Dermatol* 2005; 52:301-311.

Rogers NE, Avram MR. Medical treatments for male and female pattern hair loss. *J Am Acad Dermatol* 2008; 59:547-566.

Palmer BF. Managing hyperkalemia caused by inhibitors of the renin-angiotensin-aldosterone system. *N Engl J Med* 2004; 351:585-592.

Keene Sharon. Polymorphisms in the Androgen Receptor Gene and Finasteride Response in Women with Androgenetic Alopecia: A Pilot Study. International Society of Hair Restoration Surgery Meeting, 18th Annual Meeting 2010.

Chapter Five

Pak JP et al. The history of hair transplantation. *Am J of Cosmetic Surg* 2008; 25 (4):231-236.

Unger WP, Unger RH. Hair transplanting: An important but often forgotten treatment for female pattern hair loss. *J Am Acad Dermatol* 2003; 49:853-860.

Reed ML. Hair transplantation. In: Thorne, CH. editor. *Grabb and Smith's Plastic Surgery*, 6th Edition. 2007. p.562-572.

www.michaelreedmd.com. Live surgery. Accessed 7/09.

Chapter Six

Sinclair R. Chronic telogen effluvium: A study of 5 patients over 7 years. *J Am Acad Dermatol* 2005; 52(2):S12-S16.

Chapter Seven

Garg S, Messenger AG. Alopecia areata: evidenced-based treatments. *Semin Cutan Med Surg* 2009; 28:15-18.

Ehrmann DA. Polycystic ovary syndrome. *N Engl J Med* 2005; 352:1223-1236.

Ackerman AB et al. "Hot comb alopecia"/ "Follicular degeneration syndrome" in African-American women is traction alopecia! *Dermatopathology: Practical & Conceptual* 2000; 6(4):320-326.

McMichael A. Ethnic hair update: Past and present. *J Am Acad Dermatol* 2003; 48(6):S127-S133.

Rosenborough IE, McMichael AJ. Hair care practices in African-American patients. *Semin Cutan Med Surg* 2009; 28:103-108.

Fu JM, Price VH. Approach to hair loss in women of color. *Semin Cutan Med Surg* 2009; 28:109-114.

Assouly P, Reygagne P. Lichen planopilaris: Update on diagnosis and treatment. *Semin Cutan Med Surg* 2009; 28:3-10.

Ross EK. et al. Update on primary cicatricial alopecias. *J Am Acad Dermatol* 2005; 53:1-37.

Cheng AS, Bayliss SJ. The genetics of hair shaft disorders. *J Am Acad Dermatol* 2008; 59:1-22.

Antaya RJ et al. Short anagen syndrome. *J Am Acad Dermatol* 2005; 53: S130-S134.

Price VH, Gummer CL. Loose anagen syndrome. *J Am Acad Dermatol* 1989; 20(2): 249-256.

Koo JYM. et al. Psychodermatology. *J Am Acad Dermatol* 2000; 43:848-853.

Uno H et al. Effect of latanoprost on hair growth in the bald scalp of the stump-tailed macacque: A pilot study. *Acta Dermato-Venereologica* 2002; 82(1):7-12.

Wolf R et al. Prostaglandin analogs for hair growth: Great expectations. *Dermatology Online Journal* 2007; 9 (3):7.

Reynolds AJ et al. Trans-gender induction of hair follicles. *Nature* 1999; 402:33-34.

Korbling M, Estrov Z. Adult stem cells for tissue repair – a new therapeutic concept? *N Engl J Med* 2003; 349:570-582.

Mirmirani Paradi, Karnik Pratima. Lichen Planopilaris Treated with a Peroxisome Proliferator-Activated Receptor Agonist. Arch Dermatol 2009; 145(12) 1363-1366.